Primary Care and Dementia

Bradford Dementia Group Good Practice Guides

Under the editorship of Murna Downs, Chair in Dementia Studies at the University of Bradford, this series constitutes a set of accessible, jargon-free, evidence-based good practice guides for all those involved in the care of people with dementia and their families. The series draws together a range of evidence including the experience of people with dementia and their families, practice wisdom, and research and scholarship to promote quality of life and quality of care.

Bradford Dementia Group offer undergraduate and post graduate degrees in dementia studies and short courses in person-centred care and Dementia Care Mapping, alongside study days in contemporary topics. Information about these can be found on www.bradford.ac.uk/acad/health/dementia.Drug Treatments and Dementia

Bradford Dementia Group Good Practice Guides

Primary Care and Dementia

Steve Iliffe and Vari Drennan

Foreword by Murna Downs

Jessica Kingsley Publishers
London and Philadelphia

First published in the United Kingdom in 2001 by
by Jessica Kingsley Publishers
116 Pentonville Road
London N1 9JB, UK
and
400 Market Street, Suite 400
Philadelphia, PA 19106, USA

www.jkp.com

Copyright © Steve Illife and Vari Drennan 2001
Foreword © Murna Downs
Printed digitally since 2009

Library of Congress Cataloging in Publication Data
A CIP catalog record for this book is available from the Library of Congress

British Library Cataloguing in Publication Data
A CIP catalogue record for this book is available from the British Library

ISBN 978 1 85302 997 4

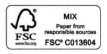

Contents

Figures

Tables

Boxes

Foreword

The National Service Framework stresses the need for effective diagnosis, treatment and support for older people with dementia and their carers. The primary care team will form a pivotal part in the achievement of these aims. GPs and allied professionals have a critical role in ensuring early identification, adequate assessment, ongoing support and timely, appropriate interventions for people with dementia and their families.

Primary Care and Dementia provides guidance on assessing and treating the whole person and not only covers ongoing medical care of people with dementia but also addresses the emotional and relationship aspects of living with the condition. The book draws on the authors' expert knowledge of the day-to-day workings of primary care to provide an accessible presentation of contemporary best practice with people with dementia for novice and experienced medical practitioners alike. There could be no better time to welcome you to this book.

Murna Downs
July 2001

This day is mine
I've yet to know tomorrow
I'll use it well
For who can tell
If joy will come or sorrow.
What was can be no more
What is can be today
I'll use the day for all its worth
Before it too will fade away.   **(Helen 1994)**

*Written by a 69-year-old woman who was
diagnosed as having Alzheimer's disease six years previously*

*Page 28 in Hearing the Voice of People
with Dementia: Opportunities and Obstacles
by Malcolm Goldsmith, 1996, Jessica Kingsley Publishers, London*

Preface

This book has been written as a guide to action. We hope it will help general practitioners and their primary health care team colleagues to:

- achieve earlier identification of dementia, to help the patient and carer come to terms with diagnosis and prognosis, to create opportunities for medical treatment and to mobilise support
- reach the correct diagnosis and detect any remedial pathology
- assess the patient's functional state and encourage optimum functioning
- trigger the provision of social support and make appropriate referrals to other agencies
- appreciate the needs of patients and carers, enabling the primary health care team to make collaborative plans for future service provision
- use medication for behaviour problems in dementia appropriately
- anticipate and avert crises
- understand the needs of carers and find ways of providing them with information, support and advice
- develop professional education programmes about the recognition of and response to dementia that meet the needs of practitioners
- commission services for dementia, and avoid the pitfalls of commissioning.

The book deliberately simplifies complex issues, so that practitioners can begin to work and reflect on complex real-life problems and find their own solutions to them. We have no easy answers. All we aim to do is outline the obstacles to good practice in dementia care in the community, and suggest some ways round them. We have based the guide on case histories rather than a recitation of evidence, because we know that most learning arises from experience more than from formal knowledge. This does not mean that we reject evidence-based practice, but rather that we know the limits to formally presented evidence and the power of problem-solving creativity among practitioners of all disciplines and among carers. Dementia is difficult to see, to understand and to experience, so we have concentrated on recognition of it, accommodation to it and action on it as the key work for practitioners.

Chapters One and Two review the problems of recognition, and the need to work towards a diagnosis that can be shared with the individual and the family. In Chapter Three we begin to describe the ways in which dementia affects individuals and families, and this theme is returned to in Chapter Five, at the end of the illness process. In Chapter Four we concentrate on the role and experience of carers, and how primary care professionals can support them. Finally, in Chapter Six we move from the perspective of the individual to the planning of education and the commissioning of local services for dementia care in the community.

We are grateful for inspiration from colleagues working on the educational and training project funded by the Alzheimer's Society and based at University College London, Stirling University and the University of Bradford, among others. Any errors of judgement or interpretation are ours alone.

Steve Iliffe
Vari Drennan
Department of Primary Care and Population Sciences
Royal Free & UCL Medical School, London

CHAPTER ONE

The Clinical Features of Dementia

INTRODUCTION

Walter A worked as long as he could, reluctantly agreeing to be pensioned off from his last job in a light engineering company at the age of 72. He pottered about at home while his wife – who was much younger – carried on with her job as a shop assistant for a few years more. He had always been a difficult character, sometimes prone to arguments but often quiet and unforthcoming. It is not clear how he spent his days, but they seemed to pass pleasantly enough, except for outbursts of irritability usually directed at his boisterous grandchildren, who renamed him 'grumpy Gramps'. Often he would sit on a stool in the kitchen doorway, looking out on to his tiny south-facing garden that caught the sun all day, and he seemed content.

Although he had proudly given up smoking in his sixties, his physical health slowly worsened, and he did less and less. From time to time his wife, now retired herself, called their GP to see him because he had taken to his bed. The doctor was jolly and called him 'Pop', and Pop always smiled and complied with whatever examination or treatment was required, but he never returned to his previous state of health.

A major change occurred when a younger relative died suddenly and tragically. Walter A wept uncontrollably for hours almost every day, his melancholy being triggered not only by any mention of the dead person, but also by words in conversations or television images that others thought unconnected to the family's sorrow. He became less able to care for himself, eventually staying in bed most of the time. When he became incontinent of faeces his exasperated wife called the GP once again, and Walter was admitted to the local cottage hospital. In a ward shared by old men with enlarged prostates and bad chests, and young men recovering from hernia operations, he was shuffled around by kindly fellow patients but forgot his family's names. Lying in bed he would pluck at the sheets with a look of alarm on his face, and at night he often called for his first wife, who had died in the influenza pandemic after the First World War.

Just after his 79th birthday he developed pneumonia, and very quickly died. At his small funeral he was said to have died of old age.

Dementia not only increases in prevalence with age (Hofman *et al.* 1991) but is also a progressive disease process with a community-wide impact (Gallo, Franch and Reichel 1991) and an unremitting course that challenges the diagnostic, management and support skills of primary care workers. In the middle decades of the last century the dementias were poorly understood and few general practitioners had an interest in their diagnosis and management, but the progressive ageing of the population has made the prevalence and incidence of dementia an issue for primary care. About 5 per cent of people aged 65 and over have some form of dementia, with the prevalence rising to about 20 per cent by 80 years and nearer one in three by 90 years. Dementia is the fourth commonest cause of death in the 75-and-over age group age group (Gray and Fenn 1993). A general practitioner with a list of 2000 patients and an average age distribution will see one or two new cases per year, have up to 14 patients with dementia at different stages of the disease process, and will carry out 70 per cent of consultations with these patients in their homes, or in residential institutions. A district nursing team with a caseload of 80 patients will typically have between 5 and 15 individuals with dementia among them. Many of these individuals will be cared for by family members or neighbours whose own health may suffer from the prolonged and difficult work of caring.

Dementia is also a huge economic burden for the community (Wimo, Ljunggren and Winblad 1997). The estimated annual cost of dementia in the UK, for example, is £5.5 billion, of which three-fifths is borne by patients, carers and social security funds, one-fifth by social services and one-fifth by the health service (Bosanquet, May and Johnson 1998). Dementia matters for families whose ageing parents and grandparents become increasingly likely to develop its early signs and symptoms, for primary care practitioners who need to understand and respond to it, and for local health and social services, which must allocate personnel, resources and training time to manage the consequences of this disease process. Everyone concerned – citizens, professionals and service managers – must adapt to the demographic changes under way and acquire the expertise needed to recognize and respond to dementia. This chapter is concerned with the recognition of the different forms of dementia, remembering Walter A, whose probable vascular dementia was never named.

Dementia is much misunderstood, and its diagnosis and management are a challenge in primary care. At the beginning memory deficits and other changes in cognition, behaviour or mood (including some features of depression) may be attributed to old age. The personality may begin to change, with emotional liability, disinhibition and sometimes verbal or even physical aggression emerging. Functional losses can appear before evident memory loss, so that individuals cannot remember which medicines to take, or how to make a telephone call. As the dementing process proceeds, awareness of memory or other problems with cognition diminishes, so the patient becomes a less reliable witness. As a consequence, relatives' complaints about the memory of a family member are suggestive of dementia, whereas complaints of memory loss made by the patient suggest depression rather than dementia. However, there is no classic presentation, since one in three patients with dementia will also have features of either a depressive disorder, or symptoms attributable to bereavement, or generalized anxiety, or an alcohol problem.

Later in the disease process higher mental functions are lost, so that the affected individuals suffer disorientation and loss of comprehension, lose the ability to calculate, and lack learning capacity, language and judgement. In the last phases of dementia the individual loses almost all functional capacity, often becomes incontinent of urine and faeces, and may be unable to communicate with others in any way. Table 1.1 summarizes the clinical features of dementia at the beginning and towards the end of its course. However, an individual's pathway through dementia is unique and influenced by their previous life experience and their social and family relationships. Some of these changes may not appear in the order listed in Table 1.1, and some may not appear at all.

Changes in the thinking, mood or everyday behaviour of an individual should prompt two questions. Could this be a form of dementia, or is there some other process at work? And, if dementia is a possibility, which type could it be? Neither question is easy to answer, but the answers are important because they shape the responses that professionals can make, and the information that they begin to share. The next section of this chapter will review the diagnosis of dementia, and its subtypes.

Table 1.1 Features of dementia at different points in its path

	Early changes	Later changes
Emotional changes	Shallowness of mood, frustration Lack of emotional responsiveness and consideration of others Depression and/or anxiety	Irritability and hostility Aggression
Cognitive changes	Short-term memory deficit with particular difficulty in registration and recall of new information Thinking becomes concrete with a reduced range of concerns Perseveration of thoughts and actions, accompanied by repetitive speech	Language disorder; both receptive and expressive dysphasia can occur Thought process becomes fragmented, so that speech becomes disordered and fragmented Psychotic features occur in 30–40% Persecutory ideas and delusions Auditory and visual hallucinations – not mood congruent
Behavioural changes	Social withdrawal Emotional and physical disinhibition Difficulty in carrying out purposeful tasks: domestic tasks, dressing, etc. Socially inappropriate behaviour, self-neglect Disorientation progressively for time, place and eventually for person	Wandering and restlessness Evening and nocturnal restlessness prominent Turning night into day Aggression and violence

Physical changes	Usually later in the disease process	Weight loss, self-neglect
		Malnutrition
		Incontinence
		Receptive and expressive dysphasia
		Bradykinesia and tremor
		Epileptiform seizures (usually late)
		Emergence of primitive reflexes
		Rigidity (usually late)
		Instability
		Visuospatial problems – less able to compensate for physical disabilities
		Immobility

Reproduced with permission from **Dementia Tutorial: Diagnosis and Management in Primary Care. A Primary Care Based Education/Research Project**. Bradford University, Stirling University and Royal Free & UCL Medical School

DIFFERENTIATING ACUTE CONFUSION, DEPRESSION AND DEMENTIA

Distinguishing dementia from other changes in thinking and behaviour that can occur at different stages of life is not a simple task, especially in the early stages of the process. The timescale of changes is important, as is the pattern of symptoms.

Dementia is a long-term disorder with a gradual onset, unlike the sudden onset of confusional states due to infection or medication side-effects. At the beginning it may be hard to distinguish from depression, which may produce memory loss, inability to carry out usual tasks, and apathy. Table 1.2 gives a rough guide to the differences between dementia, acute confusion and depression.

Table 1.2 The differential diagnosis of dementia, acute confusion and depression

	Dementia	Acute confusional state	Depression
Onset	insidious	acute	gradual
Duration	months/years	hours/days/weeks sometimes	weeks/months
Course	stable and progressive vascular dementia: usually stepwise	fluctuates: worse at night, lucid periods	usually worse in the morning, improves as day goes on
Alertness	usually normal	fluctuates	normal
Orientation	may be normal but usually impaired for time/place	always impaired: time/place/person	usually normal
Memory	impaired recent and sometimes remote memory	recent impaired	recent may be impaired, remote intact
Thoughts	slowed reduced interests perseveration	often paranoid and grandiose, sometimes with bizarre ideas and topics	usually slowed, preoccupied by sad and hopeless thoughts
Perception	normal hallucinations in 30–40% (often visual)	visual and auditory hallucinations common	mood-congruent auditory hallucinations in 20%
Emotions	shallow, apathetic, labile, irritable, careless	irritable, aggressive, fearful	flat, unresponsive or sad and fearful, may be irritable
Sleep	often disturbed, nocturnal wandering common, nocturnal confusion	nocturnal confusion	early morning wakening
Other features		other physical disease may not be obvious	past history of mood disorder

Reproduced with permission from *Dementia Tutorial: Diagnosis and Management in Primary Care. A Primary Care Based Education/Research Project*. Bradford University, Stirling University and Royal Free & UCL Medical School

Acute confusion

The development of an acute confusional state characteristically takes place over hours or days and is usually accompanied by signs of physical ill health such as infection or drug toxicity. The course generally fluctuates and is worse at night, with lucid spells occurring during the day. The level of alertness fluctuates and the person is often disoriented for time and place, though not often for person. Short-term memory is always impaired but this is a function of the confusion and lack of attention and always resolves fully.

The person is usually fearful, irritable and may be aggressive. Paranoid ideas, and visual or auditory hallucinations are common. Look for signs of chest infection and urinary tract infection, and always check medication taken. All symptoms will resolve with treatment of the underlying cause, unless the acute confusional state is superimposed on an underlying dementia.

Depression and dementia

A depressive illness in later life may be difficult to distinguish from dementia, but there are several key features which aid correct diagnosis. Look for five or more indicators from the following list which have been present for a two-week period and which affect everyday functioning:

- depressed mood most of the day
- loss of interest and/or pleasure
- significant change in weight
- insomnia or hypersomnia
- psychomotor agitation or retardation
- fatigue
- feelings of worthlessness

- concentration difficulties

- recurrent thoughts of death or suicidal ideas

- multiple physical symptoms.

The development and expression of these symptoms may occur over weeks or months but the process is usually shorter than the onset of a dementia syndrome, which may emerge over months or years. Patients with dementia tend not to complain about physical symptoms, even when they have disabling problems like extensive osteoarthritis that should produce them; and multiple somatic complaints without obvious physical cause can be a sign of depression. Sometimes the diagnosis is very difficult to make and a trial of antidepressants is the only way to differentiate finally between the two.

Depression and dementia can co-exist in up to 40 per cent of individuals with cognitive impairment, occurring mostly in the early stages of the dementing process. Treatment of the depression seems to be effective, in terms of restoring some function and reducing psychological distress, in up to 85 per cent of those with both disorders.

Sybil B had visited her GP many times in the previous two years, complaining of aches and pains in different parts, but no cause had ever been found apart from some osteoarthritis in the lower spine. Her doctor thought she was relatively fit for her 80 years, and said so. He felt irritated by her repeated visits and seemingly groundless complaints, and she felt that she was not being taken seriously. Then she began to complain about her memory loss, describing how she would put things down in her flat and not remember where they were, or forget appointments, or come home from the high street without an important piece of shopping. He tested her memory and reasoning ability with the Mini Mental State Examination (see page 38), and she scored 27 out of 30, forgetting two things and failing to copy a diagram accurately. As part of the MMSE she had to write a sentence, and she wrote 'I am depressed and need help'.

Test your own ability to distinguish dementia from other causes of confusion with these cases. The answers to the questions at the end of each case can be found at the end of the chapter.

CASE STUDY 1

Joan C, aged 78, is referred to you with a six- to nine-month history of increasing forgetfulness and confusion, aggressive behaviour, and urinary incontinence over the past two months. The family are also complaining that she lacks interest in her normal activities. She has previously been well, with no past medical or psychiatric history of note. She is not taking medication. She was widowed five years ago.

You visit her at home in the company of her son, with whom she has a supportive and caring relationship. The son lays particular emphasis on his mother's irritability and aggressive behaviour, coupled with a lack of interest in her normal activities. The son thinks that Mrs C is incontinent due to lack of will rather than lack of awareness and notes that when she visits his house she seems more motivated and is not incontinent.

Mrs C complains of feeling low and irritable, saying that she sees no point in living now that her memory is going and that she is on her own. During the following discussion, she complains of difficulty getting to sleep and of waking in the early hours of the morning, around 2 or 3am. She says she feels worse in the mornings and has a feeling of gloom and hopelessness that she cannot shake off, no matter what she does. She also lacks energy – even going to the kitchen to make a cup of tea is too much effort.

There appear to be no clear precipitants to this change in health.

On examination Mrs C is slightly dishevelled, and speaks slowly in a monotone. She is apathetic and replies to most questions with 'I don't know'. On cognitive testing she scores 26/30 on the Mini Mental State Examination, being unable to recall three words after a minute and not knowing the date. Her concentration is clearly impaired.

Does Joan have:

- early dementia?

- a depressive illness?

- acute confusional state?

- another cause for dementia-like presentation?

Turn to page 33 for the answers.

CASE STUDY 2

Mrs D is worried about her husband's increasing vagueness and forgetfulness, and has made an appointment for them both to see you at the end of surgery. Mr and Mrs D are both 63 years old. You know that the family have recently moved to your area, since taking early retirement two years ago, and now run a guest house. Alfred D has insulin-dependent diabetes with good control, and you see him regularly to review this. The last time you saw him was about a month ago when you noticed nothing wrong.

You are struck by Mr D's slightly vacant expression. He displays lack of concern about the situation but is prepared to accept that if his wife tells him something is wrong then it probably is. He is quite willing for you to see his wife again and to discuss further investigations.

Mrs D explains her anxieties about her husband in more detail. She says that he has been forgetting to note down bookings for their guest house, is not remembering telephone messages, and has difficulty in remembering items guests ask for at breakfast. He has also been forgetting personal information. For example, he forgot their wedding anniversary recently, and when Mrs D expressed her hurt, he was uncharacteristically quite unconcerned. He was also unconcerned about the birth of their second daughter's baby, although her last three pregnancies had ended in miscarriages. He was becoming increasingly vague, had become less affectionate towards her and their daughters and seemed to have no interest in the physical side of their relationship. He was anxious in social situations and had become withdrawn.

The history has become clearer and problems with Mr D's short-term memory seem to be the most pressing concern to address. You ask Mr D if anyone in his family has ever had similar problems, but he does not think so.

Does Alfred have:

- early dementia?

- a depressive illness?

- acute confusional state?

- another cause for dementia-like presentation?

Turn to page 34 for the answers.

CASE STUDY 3

George E is 86 years old and lives alone. He has had no contact with you for the past few months, having been reasonably well and only requiring repeat prescriptions. He has no previous psychiatric history. His past medical history includes hypertension and angina, very high alcohol consumption and peptic ulceration. His medication comprises GTN spray, atenolol, ranitidine and temazepam. Mr E's son, who lives nearby, and a neighbour have contacted you. They say he has become confused, paranoid and aggressive, accusing his neighbour of trying to steal his possessions, shouting abuse and threatening him. He has been turning night into day and has been wandering in the streets, partly clothed.

The son has noticed that his father is drowsy at times and is often asleep when he calls. He doubts whether his father is going to bed. He has noticed a deterioration in his father's self-care, that he has become very muddled and irritable, and also thinks he has been 'seeing things'. At the consultation Mr E is paranoid, with rambling speech and fragmented thinking, poor concentration and a fluctuating level of consciousness. He is irritable and aggressive and is disoriented in time and place, believing it to be 1944 and in the middle of a Nazi invasion. He appears to be more troubled by these experiences at night, but seems to have been well until about a week previously.

On closer questioning, it becomes clear that he had decided to give up drinking (average intake: three to five pints per night, though it had been more in the past) about two weeks ago. He had been feeling irritable and had suffered insomnia, so had increased his intake of temazepam considerably, running out about a week ago.

Does George E have:

- early dementia?

- a major depression with psychotic features?

- acute confusional state?

- another cause for dementia-like presentation?

Turn to page 34 for the answers.

TYPES OF DEMENTIA

The next step in differentiating between dementia and other causes of confusion is to appreciate the peculiarities of the different types of dementia, and what the implications of these peculiarities for treatment and care may be. There are three types of dementia:

- Alzheimer's disease

- vascular dementia

- Lewy body dementia.

Alzheimer's disease is a neuro-degenerative disorder with generalized brain cell loss, especially in the cortex, plus extracellular degenerative plaques, intracellular neurofibrillary tangles and widespread loss of cholinergic neurotransmitters. Its onset is usually over the age of 45 years and it has a progressive, unremitting course with 'global deterioration' – a widespread loss of functions and abilities. Alzheimer's disease is slightly commoner in women than in men. The definitive diagnosis is only made at post mortem, although CT scanning can show typical cerebral changes.

In vascular dementia small or large vascular lesions cause focal damage in the brain. Its onset is usually over the age of 45 years and often sudden, with focal neurological signs. It is more common in men than in women, and there is usually past history of cardiovascular pathology (particularly hypertension), plus an association with smoking. Stepwise deterioration in cognitive and physical function occurs, with uneven changes in skills and personality.

Lewy body dementia is uncommon but presents with a different pattern of symptoms (see Box 1.1). Patients with Lewy body dementia should not be treated with neuroleptic drugs because of a high risk of consequent acute illness and death.

BOX 1.1 LEWY BODY DEMENTIA

Clinical pattern in Lewy body dementia (symptoms in order of frequency):

- clouding of consciousness

- paranoid delusions

- complex visual hallucinations

- falls and 'collapses'

- depression symptoms

- auditory hallucinations

DIAGNOSING DEMENTIA

The possibility that the changes occurring in an individual could be due to one or other form of dementia may be only a suspicion in the mind of the general practitioner, nurse or social worker. Moving from suspicion to greater certainty can be a lengthy process sometimes lasting years, but it has a logical path, which we will outline here and review in more detail in Chapter Two. The first action is to obtain information from someone who knows the individual concerned. Their own observations, worries and hypotheses may have initiated the contact with the professional in the first place, making the task of information gathering easier, but requests for help may be less clearly formulated, as in the case of Walter A. In these situations a few carefully considered questions introduced into a conversation between professional and carer can help.

Informant history

As we shall see later, those closest to the individual with dementia do not always notice the early changes, or attribute them to other causes, like 'old age' or previous patterns of thought and behaviour. However, the description of changes in behaviour, mood or memory given by other family members can provide clues about the possibility of a dementing illness in situations where it is not at all clear at first glance what has made an individual change. Cognitive impairment is particularly associated with deterioration in four domains of daily activity, and questions should be asked about these:

1. forgetting to take long-term medication, or to keep appointments

2. difficulties using the telephone: not simply forgetting numbers, but forgetting how to make a phone call

3. problems managing money, adding up, sorting out change, or dealing with bills

4. difficulties using public transport.

Even in situations where family members have not considered the possibility of dementia, discussing these symptoms and signs may prompt their diagnostic thinking as well as your own, so that their awareness changes. Of course, in an increasingly knowledgeable society in which dementia has a rising public profile the prospect of this condition developing is more often in the minds of older people themselves, and of their peers and children. Nevertheless, the early changes in dementia may well be overlooked or misattributed, with a consequent delay in diagnosis, and the reasons for such delays need to be understood. We shall discuss this problem later, but first look at Figure 1.1, which attempts to summarize the diagnostic process that is needed to confirm the suspicion that the symptoms and problems an individual has could be due to one form of dementia or another.

The preceding description of the onset and the course of dementia syndromes shows how difficult it can be for practitioners in any discipline to recognize the early changes – and even some of the later ones – for what they are. We will end this chapter by considering the obstacles to recognizing dementia, and in the next chapter we will discuss some ways of overcoming these obstacles.

Delayed diagnosis

We know that dementia remains underdetected and suboptimally managed in primary care (O'Connor *et al.* 1988). For example, in nine general practices in one community study in north London only 18 per cent of those aged 75 and over and found to have MMSE scores suggesting possible or probable dementia had a diagnosis of dementia, or anything suggesting cognitive impairment, in their medical records (Iliffe *et al.* 1990). This appears to be an international phenomenon, there being wide variations in knowledge about dementia among general practitioners (Ineichen 1994; Olafsdottir and Marcusson 1996; Rubin, Glasser and Werckle 1987), with memory impairment being recognized more often than functional loss or behaviour change as an important symptom (Brodaty *et al.* 1994).

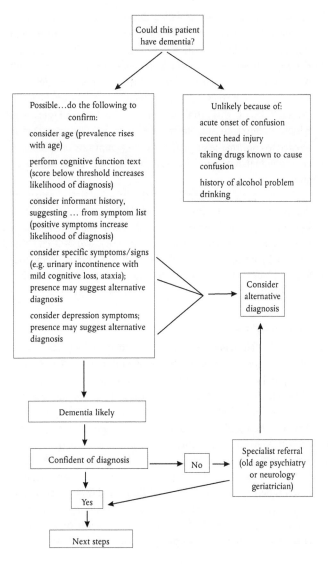

Figure 1.1 Summary of diagnostic process

Why is dementia so poorly understood, and so often poorly managed, in the community? There appears to be a large number of factors intrinsic to medical science and practice, including:

- a focus in the scientific literature (particularly in systematic reviews) upon prescribing and preventive medicine, and only on selected chronic diseases (like asthma and diabetes)

- the relative neglect of research on health and illness in older people, and the research bias towards physical rather than mental health issues

- the complexity of dementia as a psycho-socio-biological disorder, both in its lack of certain aetiology and pathophysiology, and in its high variability in symptoms and signs (De Lepeleire and Heyrman 1999)

- the absence of certainty factors, like validated diagnostic tests or monitoring measures equivalent to blood pressure, glycosylated haemoglobin or peak flow rate (De Lepeleire and Heyrman 1999)

- the limited nature of professional training in disorders of later life in the current generations of general practitioners (Alzheimer's Disease Society 1995)

- the limited qualitative research evidence available about barriers to considering, diagnosing and treating dementia.

This complexity means that the changes of dementia may be attributed to other causes, especially early in the illness. Patients with early dementia may not be recognized as having a problem for a considerable period: the time between first-noted symptoms by patient or carer and medical evaluation for dementia is on average 30 months (Haley, Clair and Saulsberry

1992). The reasons for this are multiple and complex. Individuals with cognitive impairment may attribute symptoms such as memory loss to their age (Pollitt 1996), and their carers may also accept some of the early features of dementia, like cognitive changes, functional loss or emotional lability as part of ageing. Carers may not tackle the issue out of respect for their spouse or parent (Antonelli Incalzi *et al.* 1992). Negative attitudes to ageing itself may also affect recognition and presentation of early dementia to primary care staff, and feelings of shame, guilt and incompetence in the affected individual or their family may impede help-seeking.

Education matters; so that those from higher socio-economic groups are more likely to seek medical attention earlier, and cultural background may influence early detection (Pollitt 1996). Ethnicity matters; dementia in ethnic minority elders may be particularly neglected, given the cultural factors inhibiting recognition (Rait and Burns 1998) and the dearth of research into the mental health of older people from ethnic minorities (Rait, Burns and Chew 1996), as well as the impact of language difficulties and lower educational attainment in interpreting rating scales (Escobar *et al.* 1986). The expression of problems and symptoms is culturally determined, with great variations in the expression or suppression of experiences. The attribution of symbolic meaning to symptoms and the labelling of distress or deviant behaviour as voluntary or accidental also varies greatly (Kirmayer 1989). Lack of awareness or insight, or denial, may account for some late presentation of dementia (Verhey *et al.* 1995); in one study nearly half of all patients were unaware that they had a problem at first contact (Newens, Forster and Kay 1994). Nevertheless, informant histories are crucial to investigating the suspicion of dementia, and carers may be the first to reach the diagnosis (O'Connor *et al.* 1989), even if they do not voice it or act upon it.

General practitioners and dementia recognition

Diagnoses are made in general practice through pattern recognition over time, with particular symptoms or problems described by the patient or carer triggering an iterative process of hypothesis testing that is very different from the linearity of algorithms (De Lepeleire and Heyrman 1999). The overall ability of GPs to recognize dementia is moderately good, with positive predictive values for GP diagnoses against gold standards like CAMDEX ranging from 32 per cent to 79 per cent in seven studies reviewed by van Hout (van Hout 1999). Clearly there is considerable scope for improvement, but unless primary care professionals are aware of the early signs of dementia they are unlikely to begin the diagnostic process (Lagay, van der Meij and Hijmans 1992). As already noted, loss of function may be the earliest change in many patients with dementia, and diminished capacity to use the telephone, manage medication or money, and use transport have strong predictive value for the imminent onset of dementia (Barberger-Gateau, Dartigues and Letenneur 1993), but GPs tend to associate dementia primarily with memory loss (De Lepeleire, Heyrman and Buntinx 1998).

Low awareness of the different ways dementia can present, and of available effective interventions, may be due to a limited understanding about ageing generally and dementia in particular (Alzheimer's Disease Society 1995). This probably reflects the biases of undergraduate education as well as the negative image of ageing in our culture.

The triggers that start the process of recognition of dementia are commonly:

- important functional changes, like not taking prescribed medication regularly

- behavioural disturbances, like wandering or acting in a disinhibited way

- major loss of memory, like losing the way home from the shops

- other cognitive and mood changes, like the expression of paranoid ideas

- crises – the revelatory moments when the spouse who has compensated so long for the failing memory or ability of their dementing partner has a stroke, or fractures their femur, and is admitted to hospital.

These changes may have an impact on family economics, making someone miss work, and force family members to review their own explanations for the changes in the affected person. In these situations both family members and professionals who have known the affected individual for some time may respond to the recognition of dementia with:

- disbelief that such a process is under way in the individual

- denial that the problem is dementia, sometimes with a search for another, more tolerable, explanation

- apprehension at the level of support that will be required for the individual and those around him or her

- fear of the illness.

We should not underestimate the impact of awareness of dementia as a possibility or a probability on how individuals think about themselves and others. For professionals dementia is sometimes a 'heartsink' diagnosis, but there are positive steps to take, which we will summarize here:

- exclude treatable causes like hyperthyroidism and B12 deficiency

- exclude overlapping conditions – for example depression, acute confusional state and psychotic symptoms, and concurrent physical illnesses

- minimize associated disabilities

- refer to consultant colleagues if the diagnosis is in doubt or to access additional resources

- act as the gateway to other resources

- help carers to care: provide information and advice, especially about the emotional and behavioural changes which have already taken place, or will take place as the illness progresses

- direct people to voluntary organizations for additional help.

At first sight this may seem like a formidable workload, but it is less of a problem in practice because activities are spread over time and between different professionals and organizations. These steps will be described in more detail in the following chapters.

ANSWERS TO TEST CASES
Case study 1 Joan C

The most likely answer is a depressive illness, because she has so many features of depression, including sleep disturbance, irritability and loss of energy. Early dementia, or another cause for dementia-like presentation, is less likely, but the urinary incontinence is puzzling, even for severe depression, so review this. The timescale of change makes an acute confusional state very unlikely.

Case study 2 Alfred D

The presenting illness is not acute, so an acute confusional state is unlikely. Early dementia is possible even if he is only 63 years old. There is no history of depression as far as you are aware, but this may be a depressive illness. You wonder about the possibility of another cause for dementia-like presentation – even a brain tumour – in view of his personality change.

Case study 3 George E

An acute confusional state is the most likely cause. Early dementia, a major depression with psychotic features, or another cause for dementia-like presentation, are unlikely, although the confusional state may have revealed a dementia process, perhaps induced by cerebral damage due to alcohol.

The confusional state is probably caused by alcohol withdrawal, increased intake of benzodiazepines and then abrupt cessation of these. The features which suggest this diagnosis are: sudden onset of paranoid thinking and behaviour disturbance, and the changes in use of alcohol and medication. Admission to hospital would be appropriate here, and communication with an old age psychiatrist or a geriatrician a sensible first step.

CHAPTER TWO

Confirming and Conveying the Diagnosis

I knew something was wrong, but I did not want this to be
seen by anyone else. I wanted to stay 'normal' but I found it
was hard. A struggle. I had to make lots of lists and keep them
in the house or car. We argued a lot because I never wanted to
go out. Scared you see. I was always terrified my wife would
find out. (A person with dementia, quoted from an interview
in Keady 1997, p.29)

How can we be sure that the changes occurring in an individual
are due to Alzheimer's disease, vascular dementia or some other
form of the disease? The simple answer is that achieving absolute
certainty in the diagnosis of dementia (along with many other
conditions) is not realistic in primary care, but that over time and
with the right approach primary care practitioners can reach the
diagnosis with a high degree of accuracy, sometimes, but not
always, without referral to specialists. In this chapter we will
discuss the diagnostic process, the limited range of investigations
that help in making the diagnosis, the issue of sharing the
diagnosis with the patient and their family, and the role of the
new anti-dementia drugs.

THE DIAGNOSTIC PROCESS

Early identification of dementia can be important for forward planning of care, for education of patients, families and professional teams, and for mobilization of resources. Also, recent therapeutic advances have renewed calls to improve detection and management of people with dementia because of some evidence of therapeutic benefit from selective use of the newer anti-dementia drugs. Even the earlier preparations like Tacrine (which is too toxic to be widely used) could be cost-neutral and save on nursing home placements, if used selectively and carefully by experienced clinicians. This emerging generation of medicines is an important issue for primary care workers, partly because of their complexity and cost, and partly because of growing public awareness of anti-dementia drugs. We will return to this theme later in this chapter.

Early diagnosis is also important because it allows for individuals and carers to be informed, and to be introduced to appropriate agencies and support networks which can relieve the disabling psychological distress that carers may experience (Levin, Sinclair and Gorbach 1989), even without the support being called upon (Briggs 1993). One of the commonest criticisms of general practitioners, and to a lesser extent of specialist services, is that they provide too little information about dementia and its consequences, with too little practical content that is helpful to patients and families. The case of Walter A, in Chapter One, might have been qualitatively different for him and for his wife if an effort had been made to reach and convey a diagnosis, and to mobilize support.

However, early identification is not an easy task, because it is not always appropriate to share suspicions or even near certainty about the diagnosis. The practitioner is left trying to find a way to discuss dementia with an affected individual or others who are not yet ready for such dialogue. This is a real dilemma for professionals, but we want to warn against overstating its size and scope, and to point instead to the widespread need for honesty and communication. We will return to the problem of breaking the news later in this chapter. First we must describe the ways in which suspicion of a dementia process can be confirmed or dismissed.

Cognitive function tests

The first practical question for primary care practitioners is how to identify dementia at an early stage. Cognitive function tests are useful adjuncts to clinical judgement and informant histories, as described in Chapter One. We must qualify this recommendation immediately, because none of the existing cognitive function tests that could be used routinely in primary care can make a diagnosis. All that they can do is add to the practitioner's existing knowledge of the patient and increase or decrease the likelihood of a diagnosis of dementia being possible. Their use is essentially as a decision support tool, in situations where there is already clinical suspicion. There is no reason to use them in the absence of clinical suspicion, except perhaps to help a discussion with the patient who comes to ask about memory loss when there seems little else in the story to suggest dementia. Widespread screening of whole populations of older people (as advocated by the 75-and-over checks in British general practice) is not appropriate, for there is little evidence to suggest that screening for cognitive impairment in asymptomatic individuals is beneficial (Eccles *et al*. 1998; Melzer *et al*. 1994).

The two most widely used cognitive function tests are the Abbreviated Mental Test Score (AMTS) and the Mini Mental State Examination (MMSE). The AMTS is quick and easy to use, and has become popular in hospital care because of its user friendliness, but does not give as much information as the MMSE. This test is longer to use, although this becomes less of a problem with practice, and it tests a wider range of functions, like calculation and writing skills. A less widely used but promising cognitive function test is the 6-item Cognitive Impairment Test (6CIT).

BOX 2.1 THE ABBREVIATED TEST SCORE

This is a quick and easy test that can be used in the consultation

Each correct answer scores 1 point

1. Age ☐

2. Time to nearest hour ☐

3. An address – for example 42 West Street – to be repeated by the patient at the end of the test ☐

4. Year ☐

5. Name of hospital, residential institution or home address, depending on where the patient is situated ☐

6. Recognition of two persons – for example, doctor, nurse, home help, etc. ☐

7. Date of birth ☐

8. Year First World War started ☐

9. Name of present monarch ☐

10. Count backwards from 20 to 1 ☐

Total score ——

A score of less than 6 suggests dementia

If you think someone has dementia:

- Use the abbreviated mental test score (above). This is only a rough guide to diagnosis.
- Carry out routine blood tests.

If in doubt, refer to specialist – a general psychiatrist, old age psychiatrist or neurologist depending on age of patient and who is available locally.

If diagnosis is confirmed· encourage the carer to join the Alzheimer's Society or Alzheimer Scotland – Action on Dementia.

Services: refer to social services for assessment.

Benefits: your patient should claim attendance allowance or disability living allowance care component and discount on their council tax bill. Provide the appropriate certificate.

Ensure follow up.

BOX 2.2 MINI MENTAL STATE EXAMINATION

The MMSE is a good instrument for assessing cognitive function, but takes up to ten minutes and cannot fit easily into a standard consultation

Orientation

> What is the (year) (season) (date) (day) (month)?
>
> Where are we: (country) (city) (part of city) (number of flat/house) (name of street)?

Registration

> Name of three objects: one second to say each
>
> Then ask the patient to name all three after you have said them.
>
> Give 1 point for each correct answer.
>
> Then repeat until he learns all three.
> Count trials and record.

Trials:

Attention and calculation

> Serial 7s. 1 point for each correct
> Stop after five answers.
>
> Alternatively, spell the word 'world' backwards.

Recall

> Ask for the three objects repeated above.
> Give 1 point for each correct.

Language

> Name a pencil and watch (2 points).
>
> Repeat the following 'No ifs, ands or buts' (1 point)
>
> Follow a three-stage command: 'Take a piece of paper in your right hand, fold it in half and put it on the floor' (3 points).
>
> Read and obey the following: 'Close your eyes' (1 point).
>
> Write a sentence (1 point).
>
> Copy a design (1 point).

Instructions for administration of the Mini Mental State Examination

Orientation

1. Ask the date. Then ask specifically for parts omitted, for example, 'Can you also tell me what season it is?' Score 1 point for each correct.

2. Ask in turn, 'Can you tell me the name of this place?' (town, country, etc.). Score 1 point for each correct.

Registration

Ask the patient if you may test his memory. Then say the names of three unrelated objects, clearly and slowly, about one second for each. After you have said all three, ask him to repeat them. This first repetition determines his score (0–3) but keep saying them until he can repeat all three, up to six trials. If he does not eventually learn all three, recall cannot be meaningfully tested.

Attention and calculation

Ask the patient to begin with 100 and count backwards by 7. Stop after five subtractions (93, 86, 79, 72, 65). Score the total number of correct answers. If the patient cannot or will not perform this task, ask him to spell the word 'world' backwards. The score is the number of letters in correct order, e.g. dlrow 5, dlowr 3.

Recall

Ask the patient if he can recall the three words you previously asked him to remember. Score 0–3.

Language

Naming: Show the patient a wrist-watch and ask him what it is. Repeat for pencil. Score 0–2.

Repetition: Ask the patient to repeat the sentence after you. Allow only one trial. Score 0 or 1.

Three-stage command: Give the patient a piece of plain blank paper and repeat the command. Score 1 point for each part correctly executed.

Reading: On a blank piece of paper, print the sentence 'Close your eyes' in letters large enough for the patient to see clearly. Ask him to read it and do what it says. Score 1 point only if he actually closes his eyes.

Writing: Give the patient a blank piece of paper and ask him to write a sentence for you. Do not dictate a sentence; it is to be written spontaneously. It must contain a subject and verb and be sensible. Correct grammar and punctuation are not necessary.

Copying: On a clean piece of paper, draw intersecting pentagons (as below), each side about 1 inch, and ask him to copy the drawing exactly as it is. All ten angles must be present and two must intersect to score 1 point. Tremor and rotation are ignored.

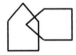

A score of 20 or less generally suggests dementia but may also be found in acute confusion, schizophrenia or severe depression. A score of less than 24 may indicate dementia in some patients who are well educated and who do not have any of the above conditions. Serial testing may be of value to demonstrate a decline in cognitive function in borderline cases.

The 6CIT is in Mentor on EMIS Mentor Plus under 'screening for dementia', and a working example of it can be found on *www.kingshill-research.org* or on *www.stjohnssurgery.co.uk/dementia*. The software is freely available and for a nominal fee can be made obtained on a CD-ROM (Brooke and Bullock 1999).

However, we must stress again that limited diagnostic skills

BOX 2.3 THE 6CIT

1. What is the date?

2. Memorize a 5-component phrase: e.g. John Brown, 42, West St., Bedford

3. What time is it? (correct to the nearest hour)

4. Count backwards from 30 to 1

5. Say the months of the year in reverse order

6. Repeat the memorized phrase (how many errors)

---

cannot be remedied by use of diagnostic instruments, which do not replicate the step-by-step approach to collecting and collating information needed to diagnose dementia (De Lepeleire, Heyrman and Buntinx 1999). For example, the limitations of brief tests like those described here may lead to a misdiagnosis of dementia, because an individual who has had only a few years of formal education, or who has significant hearing or visual loss, may perform badly on such tests (Jagger *et al.* 1992).

We need to remain cautious in using these tests for other reasons, without being nihilistic and avoiding them altogether. Dementia is a complex syndrome that emerges at an age when other morbidity may be very prominent, so a definitive test that could distinguish dementia from, say, normal forgetfulness would be valuable. Unfortunately it does not exist, at least in a form that will fit into everyday clinical practice. The absence of such a definitive test can make primary care physicians feel less confident in discussing a diagnosis, while negative attitudes to dementia or a lack of knowledge about services and interventions available may also discourage early detection.

Primary care physicians may also be concerned about the implications to patients and families of early diagnosis, and may be especially concerned about making 'false positive' diagnoses in a climate which increasingly encourages early disclosure, and when a wrong diagnosis may have significant impact on patient management (Eefsting *et al.* 1996). We know, for example, that the accuracy of general practitioners' diagnoses in a prevalence study of dementia rose significantly when a broader label of 'cognitive impairment' was used in stead of 'dementia' (*ibid.*). This uncertainty and caution about the diagnosis may even become more marked as the population learns more about Alzheimer's disease, and individuals with some element of memory loss consult their family doctor. Fortunately we can reassure the patients who do consult like this that subjective cognitive deficits in the absence of other clinical evidence of cognitive impairment do not predict the onset of dementia

(Flicker *et al.* 1993), but using a cognitive function test may be helpful to the practitioner and patient alike in reaching this conclusion.

What if a reliable, discriminating test were developed and made available to primary care practitioners? The view that the use of diagnostic instruments will solve the problem of early diagnosis is not realistic, on present evidence. On the contrary, we know that feedback of the results from cognitive function tests increases detection of mental health morbidity by primary care doctors, but has no effect on management (Shapiro *et al.* 1987). When British general practitioners used the MMSE to measure cognitive function routinely in older patients, identification of cases of possible or probable dementia did not alter the subsequent medical management of these individuals (Iliffe *et al.* 1994). It is the whole picture that matters in considering the diagnosis of dementia, not the test result.

It is hardly surprising, then, that there is no consensus on the optimal methods for diagnosing dementia in primary care (Toner 1992). Nor is it surprising that the majority of general practitioners in the UK (Ineichen 1994) and a large minority of family physicians in the USA (Fortinsky and Wasson 1997) report no use of cognitive function tests in making a diagnosis of dementia. Nevertheless we believe that using a cognitive function test – any of the ones we have described will do – when dementia is a possibility can be a useful in gaining a whole picture of the individual, and should become standard practice in primary care.

Excluding uncommon causes of dementia

If the way in which the patient explains their story, the informant's views and the results of a cognitive function test add up to a growing suspicion of dementia, what should the primary care worker do next? In a small proportion of patients with dementia there is an underlying pathology that, when treated, may result in some improvement in cognitive function – but not necessarily reversal of the dementing process. Comorbidities to exclude when investigating possible dementia are:

- hypothyroidism (and rarely so-called 'apathetic hyperthyroidism')
- B12 deficiency
- hyperglycaemia
- hypocalcaemia (from hyperparathyroidism, sarcoidosis and myeloma)
- hypercalcaemia (from metastatic cancer)
- renal failure.

Myxoedema, diabetes and B12 deficiency are not uncommon in an older population, cause a wide variety of symptoms, and are relatively easy to identify with blood testing. The minimum investigation set, requiring about 8ml of blood that can be taken at any encounter with the patient, is shown in Box 2.4, and should be documented for every person where dementia is suspected, regardless of future referral intentions. Walter A never had these tests performed and we will never know if he had any of the uncommon causes of a dementia. In retrospect it seems unlikely, since the pattern of illness fits so well with vascular dementia. In the case of Alfred D, whom we also met in Chapter One, the battery of investigations is essential.

Brain tumours are rare causes of dementia-like syndromes, as is normal-pressure hydrocephalus (in which ataxia, urinary incontinence and dementia are the classic triad of symptoms), but families and dementia support groups may want these unlikely possibilities explored and press for referral and MRI scanning. Practitioners will have to deal with these requests pragmatically, but any doubt about a particular symptom in an overall picture justifies referral for specialist reassessment.

Sotira X had never learned English in all her years in Britain, and after her husband died her son became the translator

---

BOX 2.4 MINIMUM INVESTIGATION SET

The minimum investigation list for an individual with suspected dementia should include

- a full blood count
- renal function
- TSH
- calcium levels
- blood glucose

---

who conveyed all her symptoms to her general practitioner. In her late seventies she became increasingly demanding, complaining about multiple aches and pains, and forgetting where she had left important things like her newspaper, her knitting, or her purse. Doctor and son came to agree that she was developing dementia, and assumed it was Alzheimer's type. Plans were made to involve social services to provide support for her son in home care (for he was the breadwinner) and for her personal care.

Urinary incontinence became a major problem for her, but both she and her son were very embarrassed to talk about it or for her to be examined for it, even by her very sympathetic female GP. She did agree to see a specialist in medicine for the elderly at the local hospital, who noted her unstable walk and arranged the MRI scan that demonstrated normal-pressure hydrocephalus. Surgical insertion of a shunt resulted in improved memory and amelioration (but not cure) of her urinary incontinence.

AFTER DIAGNOSIS

Once a clinical diagnosis of dementia has been reached, the next step is to assess the needs of the person with dementia and those of their carer, and to engage the relevant experts to meet those needs. It is important to recognize that your standards may not be the same as those of the patient or their carer. You need to decide what is and is not acceptable, and to balance the risks to the individual with their freedom to choose. One need may be to know as much as possible about the diagnosis and its consequences. Another may be to have the diagnosis confirmed, or to get a second opinion on it. A third may be to clarify in more detail the exact type of dementia, because of the implications for the duration of the disease process and its care. A fourth may be to have all relevant concerns about support at home discussed in detail. A fifth may be to deal with other health problems that could have an impact on the dementia, making life more difficult for the patient and their supporters. We will deal with these needs in the next sections of this chapter.

Disclosing the diagnosis

This is the task that everyone finds most difficult, but it is essential to families, carers and friends that their anxieties about dementia are dealt with directly – one of the commonest complaints heard in voluntary organizations working with dementia sufferers and their families is 'nobody told us what was happening'. In general practice we have to balance our uncertainty about the diagnosis with the need to include it as a possibility that needs investigation. Discussion of the nature of the disease process, its course and the palliative responses that can be made to it need to happen earlier rather than later, but the discussion needs to be conducted with care. Knowing the diagnosis may dispel the patient's belief that they are 'going mad', but the recognition of dementia by patient and family may result in social withdrawal, and a tendency to maximize deficits and minimize strengths and successes. Every disclosure must therefore lead on to follow-up, and to what Tom Kitwood (pioneering social psychologist) called 'positive person work' that counters the impact of neuronal losses in a realistic, accepting way.

The progressive nature of the dementias needs to be acknowledged, but not as a cruel fate against which all effort is futile. False hopes about cures or even short-term improvements are as unhelpful as saying 'there is nothing that can be done'. Equally, thinking of dementia as a 'death that leaves the body behind' neglects all the aspects of the personality that survive the decay of memory and thinking, and that can allow some people to experience relatively high levels of well-being through almost the whole course of the disease (Kitwood 1997). General practitioners who know their patients well from years of contact may be able to tailor the process of disclosing the diagnosis – or even admitting that it is one possibility – with accuracy and sensitivity, beginning the 'positive person work' at the earliest possible moment.

No one can pretend that breaking bad news is an easy task for practitioners in medicine and nursing, and each time it needs to be thought through and planned, if at all possible. The general practitioner faced with a patient with dementia has to overcome her own apprehension and fears of the disease before she can talk about it with someone equally fearful. And she also must feel reasonably sure that she will not make a bad situation worse. Avoidance of disclosure is tempting, and few doctors or nurses have not used this escape route. Some evidence of this comes from a recent postal survey of 261 GPs in Cambridgeshire, where 39 per cent reported that they always or usually disclosed such a diagnosis to patient, while over 60 per cent did not (Vassilas and Donaldson 1999). General practitioners often believe that they have little to offer dementia patients (Wolff 1994), experience explaining the diagnosis of dementia as being particularly difficult (Glosser, Wexler and Balmell 1985), and sometimes consider that giving a diagnosis does more harm than good because relatives do not want to be confronted with this reality (De Lepeleire *et al.* 1994). Studies of relatives of dementing patients report that physicians are reluctant to make a diagnosis (Haley, Clair and Saulsberry 1992; Morgan and Zhao 1993) and tend to minimize problems, while focusing on the hopeless nature of dementia (Chenoweth and Spencer 1986).

The arguments that practitioners use against the disclosure of a diagnosis to the patient, include

- uncertainty about the diagnosis and of the individual's prognosis

- lack of effective treatments, even in an age of anti-dementia drugs

- inevitability of decline

- risk of upsetting the patient and provoking anxiety.

These arguments are serious and should not be dismissed as nihilism (although they may provide camouflage for it). The counterarguments, for disclosure, need equal attention:

- Disclosure of the diagnosis relieves anxiety over symptoms noticed by patient or family.

- We all have a right to know what is happening to us.

- There is evidence that patients would wish to be told (Brotzman and Butler 1991; Maguire *et al.* 1996).

- Disclosure allows the individual and the family to make practical, legal and financial provisions.

- Recognition of the disease and its course gives an opportunity to plan future care needs and to investigate the availability of a variety of services.

The receptiveness of individuals with early dementia, and of their families, needs to be thought about while considering the best approach to disclosing the diagnosis. General practitioners may want to consider the following points:

- How will the patient understand the diagnosis and prognosis?

- What are his/her wishes about knowing?

- What are the views of the family? Is an attempt to arrive at family consensus about the diagnosis going to be helpful?

- What cultural and ethnic differences and views need to be taken into account, particularly around mental illness and truth-telling about medical conditions?

- Is there any evidence of how this person has coped with similar bad news previously?

Prior knowledge of individuals and families can be of enormous importance here, but is not available to old age psychiatrists or community psychiatric nurses coming to an individual with dementia for the first time at some point in the disease process. Whatever the benefits of specialist appraisal, the general practitioner or community nurse with background knowledge of people, families and communities has a great deal to contribute.

How should the diagnosis be given?

If a practitioner feels that the balance of the argument is in favour of sharing the diagnosis with the patient, the next question is how it should be approached. There are a number of options:

- The diagnosis could be shared over a number of consultations.

- In talking about dementia the practitioner can emphasise retained abilities and strengths, e.g. long-term memory.

- Readiness to provide information and support is conveyed by stressing availability and arranging follow-up with patients and carers.

- The practice nurse or community nurse may be able to contribute to follow-up.

- Written material can usefully supplement personal contact.

- Contact with counselling and support groups can be encouraged.

There is also evidence that the manner in which the professional discloses a serious diagnosis is important. While no guidelines on dementia developed within the profession specifically mention this, guidelines on disclosure of a cancer diagnosis (Ellis and Tattersall 1999) suggest GPs should

- explore the patient's expectations

- warn that the news is bad

- go at the patient's own pace, allowing time for the patient to react

- elicit the patient's concerns.

There is evidence from other clinical domains that presenting bad news in an unhurried, honest, balanced and empathic fashion leads to greater satisfaction with disclosure. Parents told about long-term mental or physical impairment in their infant were more likely to be satisfied with the disclosure if they felt the professional had been sympathetic, was a good communicator, and was understanding and direct (Sloper and Turner 1993).

Being given enough information, and having opportunities to ask questions were also found to be important. The seriousness of the news (in this case, the severity of the child's developmental or physical disability) did not predict parental satisfaction with disclosure. We are describing a dialogue, in which the development of a common view with the patient and family as to the nature of the problem is the first step.

Gateways to support, information and services

Criticisms of general practitioners' management of dementia include late referral to specialist and social services, often during crises, and a narrow perspective on management that posed the status quo against a single alternative of long-term institutionalization (Wright, Ball and Colemand 1988). The messages from all the literature is that the person with dementia and their family need to be in touch from the earliest point with those people who can best provide the network of support, information and services. It is very clear that there is huge variation in statutory and voluntary provision in the four countries of the UK. However, at a minimum, the general practitioner should ensure that the person with dementia and their family have gateways to people, information and services who can

- confirm the diagnosis

- help them with their psychological distress

- help them access services

- help them deal with financial and legal issues

- provide a care management framework to help detect and address changes in their needs.

So at a minimum from general practice we should aim at

- referral to specialist secondary care services for confirmation of diagnosis (in some instances) and information about the range of specialist support for people with dementia

- referral to the local personnel who can undertake detailed assessment, care planning and provision of support and services within a care management process

- recommendation of sources of information on dementia

- including details of the national Alzheimer's Society and its local branches.

Look back at the case of Alfred D (Case study 2, Chapter One) in the light of these recommendations. There is enough uncertainty about his history and symptoms to warrant referral to an old age psychiatrist or geriatrician, after doing the baseline investigations. The point of the referral is to increase certainty in clinical thinking, but the rationale for it needs to be made explicit – it is important to find out what is causing Alfred D's change in behaviour, and to see if he has one or other form of dementia. The specialist may want to exclude a rare cause of a dementia-like syndrome by doing a CT scan, and only after that investigation can the diagnosis be discussed finally. At this point both Alfred D and his wife (and other family members) may need time to discuss the implications of the diagnosis, and this time needs to be created in specialist or generalist settings. Contacting social services to arrange a social care assessment needs discussion, as does getting information and support from the local branch of the Alzheimer's Society or equivalent. The broad goals of support need to be outlined – improving cognition and daily living skills, reducing excess disability and distress, maintaining the quality of life of patient and carers, and sustaining home care.

Referral to specialist secondary care services

Are there local guidelines on when to ask for advice from old age psychiatrists, neurologists or geriatricians? In our view they can be captured in a few words. If in doubt about the diagnosis, refer. That doubt may be more on the part of the patients or members of the family, but it is no less important than that of the practitioner. Financial concerns about use of services, or the potential for prescription of expensive anti-dementia drugs, should not influence the clinical decision to seek expert reassessment and advice. In the present climate patients and carers will have anxieties about rationing and age barriers to care in their minds, even if they do not express them. Early referral to specialists services, such as memory clinics, can be helpful to all concerned, in confirming the diagnosis, helping mobilize resources, providing a new source of information and demonstrating the breadth of provision available to the individual and those around them. The difficult question may be more to do with which source of expertise to enrol than whether to seek assistance at all, and here local knowledge is crucial. In areas without an old age psychiatrist the medical choices are limited to neurologist or geriatrician, and here the special interests of the clinicians matter.

Assessment, care planning and care management

For the individual with dementia, and for those around them, the everyday tasks of life are more important than any score on a cognitive function test. Identifying problems in these abilities, problems in the coping strategies and helping the person with dementia and their family to address and plan for them is vital. The GP working with the patient and the family may be the first to share the diagnosis with them, and it may be obvious that they meet the eligibility criteria of the local authority for a full comprehensive assessment under the Community Care Act to prevent a breakdown in their present arrangements for care and support. In this situation immediate referral to the relevant social work team is required. In other situations it may be very early in the progress of the dementia when it is more appropriate to establish a baseline of abilities with a mechanism for monitoring and review, as well as to provide a source of information and support. There are different local arrangements for the provision of this second source of help. In some areas it can be provided by health visitors for older people, in others by community psychiatric nurses for older people. Some areas have specialist community nursing services (the Admiral Nursing Service) to provide both specialized care management functions, information and support to carers.

A baseline assessment of the person with dementia would include gathering information on

- the person's view of any difficulties or problems at the present

- the network of people in the daily life of the person with dementia

- household composition

- interests/social activities and pattern of a typical day

- other significant recent events, e.g. bereavements

- emotional and other mental health issues, e.g. loneliness

- the medication being taken, on prescription, bought over the counter, or borrowed from helpful friends and neighbours

- ability to communicate – speech, hearing, writing, reading, using a telephone

- ability to undertake domestic and household tasks

- mobility inside and outside the home

- sleep patterns

- diet, ability to get meals and changes in appetite

- orientation inside and outside the home

- ability to undertake personal care, e.g dressing, washing, going to the toilet

- financial/benefit issues

- balance of risks.

Not all of this information can, or necessarily should, be collected in one discussion and some of it – like financial affairs and incontinence – has to be discussed with sensitivity. Here a prior relationship with the person and their family may be more helpful than a systematic interview, and general practitioners may contribute knowledge to that gained by nurses or social workers. Nevertheless, a checklist in the medical record as well as in the community nurse's notes or the social work file would be helpful, to prompt discussion and develop a profile of needs and capabilities. Forward-thinking practitioners in these disciplines might even develop a common record, interchangeable between agencies, while the most forward thinking might expect the patient and carer to hold it.

Knowledge of the local system is vital so that the earliest referral can be made for a way into services which provide

- information and advice for the individual

- psychological support and therapy for the individual

- advice, support and training for the carer

- direct care provision

- breaks from caring for the carer

- aids, technological help and adaptations.

I feel blessed by the help and support I get. My husband was diagnosed with Alzheimer's disease five years ago. We have a marvellous team of doctors at our medical centre who gave time and advice. A few weeks after George was diagnosed I had a community nurse call at our home. Margaret now calls every two months to check George's medication and also makes arrangements to see me on my own at our local hotel. It is surprising how big problems become small over a cup of tea. (MJ, Carickfergus, Alzheimer's Society Newsletter, March 1999)

One specific issue that may be important to patient and family alike in the early phases of dementia is the value of a 'living will', or advanced directive. A living will allows an individual to record wishes about future medical and nursing care before their condition deteriorates to the point that they cannot participate in any decision-making process. A majority of older people would choose 'comfort only care' rather than active care that might leave them dependent and more disabled, although few of those interviewed know about living wills (Schiff, Rajkumar and Bulpitt 2000). American experience suggests that this is likely to change, and primary care professionals will need to know enough about living wills both to engage their patients in dialogue about them and to point them in the right direction to create one. There are problems with such anticipatory documents, which if too general will be open to interpretation, and if too specific might prescribe unworkable patterns of care; but they may be valuable planning tools that when regularly reviewed can guide the process of care. Medication use will become an increasingly important issue in dementia care, and may be a key concern in writing a living will. Few people have not heard that there are anti-dementia drugs available, and they will want to know about them.

Table 2.1 New anti-dementia drugs

DRUG	TYPE	IMPACT	RISKS	USE
Donepezil[1]	Anticholinesterase	Some improvement in cognition and global functioning in some patients, but benefits not sustained beyond six months	Liver toxicity Contra-indicated in asthma Dose-related transient diarrhoea and vomiting, fatigue, muscle cramps and dizziness	Treatment of individuals with mild to moderate Alzheimer's should be initiated by specialists and effectiveness reviewed after 12 weeks
Rivastigmine[2]	Anticholinesterase	Some improvement in cognition and global functioning in some patients	Nausea and vomiting, loss of appetite and weight, dizziness	Treatment of individuals with mild to moderate Alzheimer's should be initiated by specialists and effectiveness reviewed after 12 weeks
Galanthamine	Dual action: Anticholinesterase and acetylcholine release	Improvement in cognition, global functioning and behavioural symptoms over a 12-month period		Treatment of individuals with mild to moderate Alzheimer's should be initiated by specialists and effectiveness reviewed after 12 weeks
Traditional NSAIDs (including Aspirin)[3]	COX1 inhibitors	Potential for treating and preventing Alzheimer's disease	Gastrointestinal bleeding	Experimental only – trial results are awaited
New NSAIDs	COX2 inhibitors	Potential for treating and preventing Alzheimer's disease	No gastrointestinal tract bleeding?	Experimental only – trial results are awaited

Note

1 Burns, Russell and Page (1999); 2 Roessler et al. (1999); 3 McGeer (2000).

THE ROLE OF ANTI-DEMENTIA DRUGS

A number of new medical treatments for Alzheimer's disease have appeared since 1997, and practitioners need to be aware of them and their potential. New generations of anti-dementia drugs are likely to emerge quickly, but are likely to be used more by specialists than general practitioners, at least initially. The changes in the medication available for Alzheimer's disease make early identification of dementia, and engagement with specialist services even more important. Table 2.1 describes the mechanism, impact, risks and clinical use of three new drugs, and of widely available non-steroidal anti-inflammatory drugs In Chapter Three we will discuss medication use for behaviour problems in dementia, as part of the clinical response to the difficulties and challenges that the progression of dementia creates.

CHAPTER THREE

The Pathway of Dementia

> I had to be pushy just to get a diagnosis. The specialist we saw told us nothing except my husband had Alzheimer's Disease. He asked if I had any questions but I was too dazed to think what to ask. A few days later I had many questions but it was too late … When I left the specialist I felt utterly abandoned. No one told me what to expect when the disease became more advanced and I did not know who to turn to for help. I feel guilty for not knowing enough but we just did the best we could at the time. (JS, Norwich. Alzheimer's Society Newsletter, December 1998/January 1999)

The individual with dementia is an active person responding and adapting to the disease, rather than a passive body succumbing to pathology (Cottrell and Schulz 1993). The disease process is experienced with a unique set of perceptions and a repertoire of coping skills acquired during life. It is hardly surprising that dementia emerges in such different ways in different people, and runs such a different path, for the resourcefulness of the individual in the early stages of the disease may be unaffected and put to good use, while her uniqueness will appear differently later in the disease path, perhaps as behaviour inexplicable to those who do not know the person well enough. It is no wonder that family members and professionals alike may not recognize the early changes that occur in dementia, because they are so mixed in with the ordinary, usual, good and bad characteristics of the person. Nor is it surprising that professional and lay carers can be bewildered, frightened and distressed by behaviours that seem to them to be meaningless. We shall explore these issues in this chapter, and look at some of the responses to them.

ADJUSTING TO LOSS

The losses experienced at the beginning of dementia may provoke stages of reaction and adjustment (Cohen, Kennedy and Eisdorfer 1985), including:

- *Recognition and concern.* Mr D's wife, in Chapter One, knew the changes that were occurring in him and in his relationships with others were not part of normal ageing, and sought help.

- *Denial.* Neither Walter (Chapter One) nor his wife put any thoughts about the reasons for his slow deterioration into words or actions, except when they were unable to manage their situation unaided.

- *Anger, guilt and sadness.* These are the common emotions that emerge after the diagnosis is learned, but they may persist throughout the course of the illness and beyond.

- *Coping.* Adaptation to the impact of dementia, and the increasing demands of the person with dementia, forces family and other carers to 'get by'.

- *Maturation.* An element of acceptance and understanding in individuals with good coping strategies allows both the patient and the carers to do more than 'get by'.

- *Separation from the self.*

This last stage, the separation from the self, may be easily misunderstood as the disappearance of the self, but this view may reflect the inability of those around the affected individual to keep up with that person's changing state. Since we do not consist of memory alone but have feelings, imagination, energy, desires and will, the person with dementia can retain and express a sense of uniqueness until death, losing mostly their public or social self (Downs 1997). Professionals may be particularly affected by the loss of the social person, focusing on the illness and its problems, while family members or friends may have a stronger sense of the normality of the person with dementia. Well-supported carers rarely talk about 'personality change' or the 'loss of the person', but rather behave as if dementia represented a loss of resources, and a breakdown of defences, in the affected individual (Kitwood 1997). The person who was once over-controlled emotionally may express rage as their dementia progresses, and the individual who has been sexually inhibited may become embarrassingly disinhibited.

The wide variations in the experience of dementia reflect the wide variations in our coping styles. Those with limited insight in their earlier lives, and a restricted repertoire of psychological ideas, may pass into dementia with blame and delusions. The obsessional individual may deploy denial for long periods, while those more open to experience, with more robust defences, may not seek to blame themselves or others, nor avoid their new reality. Kitwood argues that those who have never had highly differentiated feelings – who are 'unpsychological' – are very vulnerable to dementia, for when cognition is impaired defences collapse and raw emotion is expressed.

In general practice or community nursing the knowledge that practitioners acquire about their patients, their families and the local community can help the professionals to understand the changes that are occurring within an individual with dementia. This knowledge can be conveyed to others – to the old age psychiatrist, to social care workers, or to the staff of a nursing home – who do not have the advantage of prior knowledge of the person. And it can be used to tailor support to the patient and their carers. Support and therapy for the stages of adjustment and accommodation to dementia can address one or all of the following:

1. *Mood management* – working on negative and unhelpful beliefs (in the patient and those around them) to promote adaptation may be particularly important in the denial stage.

2. *Cognitive rehabilitation* – enhancing retained cognitive strengths and developing compensatory strategies to optimizing daily functioning. Memory training, to improve the ability to recall simple information like the names of friends or neighbours, seems particularly effective if combined with instruction to caregivers on how to support the training. Reality orientation, including constant explanation, encouragement and verbal reinforcement combined with a regular daily routine plus auditory and visual clues in the environment, also improves cognitive function.

3. *Life review* – to foster integrity rather than despair in the face of a dementing process. This is the basis for reminiscence therapies.

We are not arguing that primary care workers can undertake these tasks on top of their usual work, but that they can inform the tasks when others perform them, and reinforce the processes in small ways when they are in contact with the patient and the patient's family. Brief encounters with patients and their carers can include discussions about ideas, feelings and actions that will add to the work done by others, but only if the basic approaches are held in the practitioner's mind. In that sense the role of the general practitioner, practice nurse or district nurse in dementia care is similar to the work they do with people diagnosed with one or other form of cancer. Primary care practitioners do not deliver the chemotherapy, but they know just enough about it to discuss its impact and significance. Denial, anger, guilt and sadness are emotions that appear after the diagnosis of cancer too, and we are familiar enough with them to have some responses that can support the individual, if only tangentially.

Depression revisited

Recognition of a transition from sadness to depression is one of those responses. In Chapter One we discussed the differences between depression that impairs cognition and the cognitive impairment that characterizes dementia, and we tried to show how blurred are the boundaries between these two states. We return to depression here because depression is common in people with dementia, as they experience continuing failure, and produces excess disability by adding loss of energy and interest to their cognitive decline.

Normal grief at loss takes all of us through a phase of depression, but we emerge from it. This can happen in dementia too, but there is also a tendency to become fixed in the depressed phase. Here primary care knowledge can be helpful, especially if there is a previous history of depressive illnesses or episodes. Low mood occurs more often than a major depressive illness, possibly as a reaction to the cognitive and functional changes of dementia, and attempts to improve it using one of the techniques described above would be justified. On the other hand major depression with its loss of energy, drive and pleasure is so disabling that treatment with antidepressant medication is appropriate.

We will discuss treatment options later in this chapter, but with the qualification that neither decisions about therapies nor the therapies themselves can be made easily by one practitioner alone. More often than not several different judgements are helpful.

JOINT WORKING

Care of an individual with dementia requires different disciplines to work together. A management plan is important, shared across a multidisciplinary network that includes the main carers and local voluntary organizations. This plan should include:

- *Needs assessment*, incorporating consideration of co-morbidities, mental state, difficulties with activities of daily living and behavioural problems. Such an assessment would be ideal if organized as a minimum data set that can be exchanged between disciplines. This task is a primary care responsibility, with input from social care, district nursing and community psychiatric nurses, but the common data set eludes us. Perhaps, if primary care trusts evolve to include social care, such a common record can emerge.

- *Support for carers*, including information about legal rights and responsibilities, financial help and driving. We will return to this briefly at the end of this chapter, and in more detail in Chapter Four.

- A tailored *follow up* plan, identifying a key worker and the responsibilities of other practice members. Both social care and community mental health teams have much to offer general practice here, in terms of systematised approaches to continuing care. The key worker should be the first point of contact for the patient and carer, chosen with patient and carer if possible, named and recorded in the medical and social care records, able to contact other relevant professionals and able to nominate a deputy.

- *Referral criteria* to different agencies, agreed locally, as discussed in Chapter Two.

- *Specialist input on medication use*, particularly with the new anti-dementia drugs, but also with medication prescribed for behavioural disturbance or psychotic symptoms.

BEHAVIOUR CHANGE

People with dementia can develop a range of behaviours that can be disturbed and disturbing for all concerned. Behaviour disturbances are a major source of stress for both family and professional carers, and need to be investigated carefully to tailor responses and avoid the risks of iatrogenesis. Some of the behaviours that can occur in the course of dementia are:

- repetitive questioning

- following someone around

- hiding and losing things

- walking, pacing and searching

- repetitive phrases and actions

- fidgeting or restlessness

- continual shouting of the same word or for someone, or continual screaming/wailing

- laughing or crying uncontrollably for no apparent reason

- lack of inhibition

- high levels of suspicion

- hallucinations and delusions

- aggression – verbal and/or physical.

Some of these are obviously more problematic than others – although primary health care professionals should not underestimate the effect of living with someone who continually repeats the same questions or is continually hiding, rearranging and then losing possessions. Some behaviours can be the result of multiple causation – for example, aggressive behaviour is associated with other underlying medical disorders, delusions or misidentifications, or the care setting and the attitudes of carers. In trying to understand and then address the behaviour it is important to elicit

- a clear description of the behaviour

- what led up to the behaviour, contributory factors

- who else was involved and what they were doing

- the environment it happened in

- previous occurrences of the event

- any previous interventions/actions that helped.

THE CAUSES OF BEHAVIOURAL PROBLEMS

It can be difficult to understand the origins of behavioural changes in dementia, particularly when they emerge in a crisis on a Sunday evening, unexpectedly on a house call to a patient whose dementia has not yet been recognized, or in the relatively unfamiliar environment of the nursing home. A useful mnemonic to help determine the causes of behavioural problems and how best to approach them is PAID – Physical, Activity-related, Intrinsic, and Depression or Delusion.

Physical

Physical problems can be a cause of behavioural disturbance. For example, the pain from osteoarthritis can make somebody more aggressive than usual, or they may be wandering more to attempt to relieve pain. Infections can also cause behavioural disturbances in people with dementia, and here the task is to distinguish acute confusion (see Chapter One) from chronic confusion – the revelation of a dementia process through intercurrent illness.

Activity-related

Behavioural disturbances may appear when the carer is undertaking a particular activity. For example, helping with intimate tasks like dressing or bathing may trigger aggressive responses, and in these circumstances it may be advisable for the carer to leave the room, for on their return the aggression will have dissipated. Activity-related responses can also appear when there is lack of activity – pacing up and down or repeating phrases are ways in which some people may be providing themselves with occupation.

Intrinsic to dementia

There are some behaviours intrinsic to dementia, especially, but not exclusively, in the later stages of the disorder. For example, people may wander more or repeatedly stroke another person. Unaccountable laughing or crying uncontrollably is often a feature of vascular dementia. Explaining to carers that these behaviours are intrinsic to the disorder may help them to cope with these problems.

Depression and delusions

People with delusions or hallucinatory experiences can become behaviourally disturbed. The focus for treatment should be the psychosis rather than the behavioural disturbance itself, but be cautious with medication (see below) and involve a specialist in old age psychiatry or medicine for the elderly if in doubt.

COPING WITH BEHAVIOURAL PROBLEMS

Some behaviours may result from the loss of short term memory combined with the emotional experience of the person with dementia – following behind someone asking the same questions over and over again may be the result of anxiety and insecurity. There can be ways of addressing certain questions for a while: for example, the repeated asking of 'What's today?' can be helped by having a prominently displayed clock which also has the day of the week and date. However, understanding that the underlying emotion is anxiety may need different strategies – the person with dementia may need to hear that the carer is still in the home.

Some behaviours are communication signals for particular needs. For example, fidgeting with trouser fastenings or lifting the hem of skirts may be the sign that the person with dementia needs to go to the toilet. Incontinence is a common problem. Walter A, in Chapter One, only became a problem for the health service when his wife could no longer cope with his faecal incontinence, and the response was to admit him to hospital. An earlier enquiry might have been helpful, if it had included the questions:

- What kind of incontinence and how often?

- Are there contributing factors (e.g. medication causing faecal impaction and overflow incontinence, inability to get to the toilet)?

- What means of containment are available (e.g. pads or laundry services) that would improve the quality of life of patient and carer?

Carers need to be offered ideas and support in coping with the behaviour of each individual as well as avoiding confrontation. It might be helpful, for example, to identify suitable distraction strategies for an elderly man with dementia who frequently handles his genitals, rather than using punishment such as slapping the hands away. Ideas might be offered on simple measures that could be introduced to make wandering safer, such as having contact details pinned inside all clothes and on a bracelet, or creating 'safe wandering' areas by disguising some doorways and leaving others free; those would be preferable to restraining a person with dementia into a chair with ties.

The following are some ideas for avoiding confrontation with people with dementia:

- Talk in a calm, reassuring tone at normal volume.

- Approach the person in their line of vision before talking.

- Pay attention to your and their body language – try to remain at the same physical level as them (see Chapter Five for a fuller list of suggestions on improving communication skills).

- Allow enough time to undertake conversations and activities at their pace, not yours – this may often mean not trying to do too many things one after another.

- Find ways of enhancing communication with non-verbal cues.

- Be aware if the person with dementia is physically uncomfortable (e.g. in pain, or needing to pass urine).

- Provide reassurance rather than outright denial of their fears or delusions.

- If you start getting irritated or feel angry with the person, take time out, calm down and then come back.

- If the person with dementia starts showing signs of agitation or aggression, cease what you are doing and withdraw, returning later, perhaps in the company of someone they know or trust more.

REFUSAL OF HELP

Despite all the best efforts of carers and professionals to find ways to cope with and manage the change in behaviour and loss of abilities, it is common to meet refusal or rejection of help from the person with dementia. Refusal to be helped often makes family carers and professionals distressed or worried. The questions to ask out loud are:

- How do the risks balance against the choice of the individual?

- What strategies for coping are available, and which professionals and services should be involved in thinking about risk and risk management?

- When should we review the situation?

Refusal to accept admission to residential care can be the most challenging of all, and should prompt all concerned to think:

- How can risks be limited?

- Is extra community support available?

- Are compulsory procedures appropriate?

- Can anyone be appointed guardian?

The full range of expertise may be needed to manage situations like these. The case study below follows a complex problem through to a satisfactory outcome; in Chapter Five we will discuss a situation where no such positive result is possible. Put yourself in the position of the general practitioner in this next vignette.

CASE STUDY 4

Mrs Margaret G is 82 years old and lives alone with her cat. Her only surviving family is a niece, some 35 miles away, who has little contact with her. Mrs G has been known to both her GP and social worker for some time, and her GP visits regularly. Attempts have been made over the past couple of years to persuade her to accept services but she has resolutely refused. One supportive neighbour has died and another has moved away. Mrs G has deteriorated physically over the last three to four months, has become more confused and has been wandering. A crisis has occurred because she has been disturbing her neighbours at night by pounding on the shared wall of their houses, and has developed paranoid ideas about them which she reports to the police on a regular basis. She is also very anxious and fearful, and sometimes barricades herself into her home. Mrs G has no past medical history of note and, other than her dementia, has no other psychiatric history. She has not been prescribed any medication for years. The GP has been contacted by her neighbours and social services who say 'something must be done'.

Renewed contacts

The general practitioner visits Mrs G again and notes a strong smell of urine in her home and evidence of faecal smearing. There is virtually no food in the house, apart from a few packets of biscuits. There is no obvious medical cause for her deterioration, other than a possible urinary tract infection, and she allows her doctor to take a blood sample for a routine haematological screen. She also

---

provides a urine sample but adamantly refuses offers of social support.

In a subsequent telephone conversation the GP and social worker agree that social support has broken down as a result of the loss of Mrs G's supportive neighbours. Her daily routine has disappeared, she has not been eating regularly and has become mistrustful of her new neighbours. She needs to form a trusting relationship once again but her paranoid ideas impede this, and given the state of her home she needs home help daily, at least initially. A day centre or day hospital place would enable her to have appropriate stimulation and more support and may encourage her to accept residential care in the longer term if community support is not enough. The day hospital would be a good environment to investigate further any other medical problems. The GP is strongly encouraged by the social worker to request an old age psychiatrist's opinion. The social worker is encouraged by the GP to complete comprehensive community care assessment procedures.

Next encounters
Mrs G has a urinary tract infection. The general practitioner suspects she is constipated but she will not allow rectal examination. No other physical abnormalities have been detected. The general practitioner does not think she needs urgent admission to hospital but asks the district nurse to call twice daily for a week to administer antibiotics. The district nurse has very limited success in gaining entry and persuading Mrs G to take her medication.

The old age psychiatrist is unable to add anything to the assessment of the situation but is able to offer emergency assessment at the day hospital, which Mrs G promptly refuses. The social services care manager agrees that, with considerable input, Mrs G could be supported at home. She takes a disliking to the social worker and refuses this.

The old age psychiatrist offers to ask the community psychiatric nurse to visit on a regular basis to try to form a trusting relationship and encourage her to accept others entering her house. She also suggests a small dose of Risperidone to try to reduce Mrs G's paranoid ideas. To everyone's surprise Mrs G accepts both the visits and the medication. After a couple of weeks of antipsychotic medication, she is more receptive to the idea of letting new people into the house. She has come to trust the CPN and gradually home help is started in the mornings. The situation is temporarily resolved.

The situation changes again
Three months later the general practitioner is contacted by the social worker to say that Mrs G has deteriorated further and there are more concerns regarding her safety as she has started wandering again and it is now winter. There is a real risk that she will wander at night, inadequately dressed for the weather, and get lost or injure herself. It becomes clear that her dementia has progressed to the point where she can no longer be maintained in the community. She refuses residential care in any form. Neither the general practitioner nor the old age psychiatrist feel that Margaret G is detainable under the Mental Health Act but feel that she will require admission soon and both wish to avoid emergency hospital admission in a crisis. A case conference is called; it is felt that to help her to improve her quality of life the option of residential care should be pursued sooner rather than later. Guardianship proceedings are started by the social worker involved as she requires care and protection rather than psychiatric treatment. Her niece is app-

ointed guardian and together with the now trusted CPN is able to convince Mrs G to take up a place in a residential home where she soon settles in. Her paranoid thinking and behavioural problems decrease, but she continues to wander.

THE USE AND MISUSE OF MEDICATION

Wherever possible, underlying causes for behaviour disturbance should be managed before prescribing medication. Tranquillizer use to control behaviour disturbance should not be prescribed routinely, although short-term use of neuroleptic agents may be appropriate, in crisis situations (unless Lewy body dementia is suspected). The expertise of community psychiatric nurses and old age psychiatrists is invaluable both in assessing and dealing with behaviour disorders and in deciding if and when medication may be helpful.

Medication use in dementia is controversial, because neuroleptics given for behaviour disturbance can precipitate falls and confusion without necessarily having a beneficial effect on behaviour. Antidepressants in therapeutic dosages may have a significant effect on depression symptoms in early dementia, but need to be evaluated against explicit criteria like activities of daily living, level of functioning, behaviour disturbance and biological features of recent onset. Other types of medication may also complicate the situation of the individual with dementia, as the case of Mr H shows.

There are clearly several areas to be considered in the primary care management of this man's problems. Taking a diuretic at night is not rational, is probably aggravating his nocturnal incontinence and possibly causing an electrolyte imbalance, aggravating his confusion. The solution is to change the administration of the diuretic to morning when he may be better able to cope with toileting from a physical and cognitive point of view, and also to check his creatinine and electrolyte levels.

CASE STUDY 5

Mr H has vascular dementia and has been deteriorating rapidly over the past few months. The main problems precipitating this contact were incessant wandering by day and night, intermittent aggression especially when physical interactions were taking place, and verbal aggression when his wife tried to persuade him to undertake activities. He is also incontinent of urine frequently, especially in the evenings, and has recently been incontinent of faeces and has been attempting to evacuate his rectum manually. His appetite has been poor and mealtimes are a source of friction and aggression. His sleep has also been poor. His past medical history consists of chronic renal failure and hypertension. His medication consists of bumetanide at night and haloperidol (5mg bd). Mr H is unable to give any account of his current problems, having severe receptive and expressive dysphasia. He is able to respond to social cues and is initially very pleasant and polite. But as the interview progresses, he becomes restless and begins to pace. He responds aggressively to his wife when she attempts to persuade him to sit down. His wife has noticed that since haloperidol was commenced (four weeks ago) and the dose increased (two weeks later), he has become more restless and has been pacing more, especially after the dose is given. She has noticed stiffness and difficulty in getting in and out of the bath, resulting in refusal to bathe. He also has difficulty in getting out of armchairs. He seems more sedated and less interested in his surroundings, and he is less able to be distracted by previously enjoyed activities.

Mr H has akathisia and stiffness as a result of being given haloperidol, which has become worse since the dose was increased. Constipation may also be a result of, or aggravated by, haloperidol. Here an inappropriate antipsychotic drug is being used to try to manage his aggression and restlessness, but is not being used to treat psychotic phenomena. It should be discontinued and causes for the behavioural changes should be sought, asking for help from a CPN or old age psychiatrist if necessary. If use of medication is unavoidable, either give a small dose of sedative antidepressant with few side-effects (for example, trazodone) or a more sedative antipsychotic with less propensity to cause akathisia and extra pyramidal side-effects (for example, chlorpromazine in a starting dose of perhaps 10mg tds, adjusting as necessary).

Mrs H may find it helpful to discuss with a CPN strategies to respond to the difficult behaviour and avoid confrontations. Help in dealing with the incontinence, once medical causes are excluded, could be sought from the district nurse or continence nurse specialist.

To sum up, we suggest that medication has a very limited role in managing the behavioural and psychological or psychiatric problems of dementia, with the probable exception of major depression. The low side-effect profile of the selective serotonin re-uptake inhibitors makes them a suitable choice for the drug treatment of depression, if this is judged appropriate. Agitation, aggressive behaviour or hallucinations can be reduced to some extent by use of antipsychotic medication, although the benefit with the older drugs is small and the effect is unrelated to dose or duration of treatment (Schneider, Pollock and Lyness 1990). Since there is also some evidence that continued use of neuroleptics may accelerate the pace of cognitive decline (McShane *et al.* 1997), prescribing medication for behavioural disturbances in patients with dementia should be based on specialist advice. Table 3.1 gives examples of the benefits and hazards of prescribing commonly used drugs.

Table 3.1 Prescribing for behaviour problems and psychotic symptoms in dementia

Types	Examples	Effects	Dosage	Comments
Newer antipsychotics	Risperidone, Sulpiride	A balanced dopamine/serotonin antagonist with relatively few anticholinergic or antiadrenergic side-effects. Can cause considerable sedation in the elderly but is useful in people with contra-indications to other older antipsychotics, or those with Lewy body dementia	Suggested dose: Risperidone 0.5mg bd increasing in 0.5mg to 1–2 mg bd; Sulpiride: 400–800mg in two divided doses	All of the older antipsychotics may be contra-indicated in people with Lewy body dementia, who may have extreme adverse reactions. Risperidone can cause orthostatic or hypotension and Parkinsonian symptoms. Special precautions: epilepsy, renal, hepatic and cardiovascular disease
Hypnotics	Benzodiazepines (e.g. Temazepam, Triazolam)	These can cause problems due to dependence, tolerance and hangover effects. They should only be used in the short term or as a last resort		Hypnotics should only be used with caution in patients with dementia and for a short period
	Zopiclone	This is a newer hypnotic with relatively short half-life. Only for short-term use	Dose range: 0.5mg – 6mg daily	Zopiclone acts in a similar manner to the benzodiazepines and dependence on the drug has already been reported
Antiparkinsonian medication	Anticholinergic drugs (e.g. Biperiden, Benztropine)	Such drugs can cause confusion and further impair cognition in the demented patient as well as ocular, cardiovascular and gastrointestinal malfunction		Avoid them

SUPPORT FOR THE CARER

If medication has a limited value in helping people with
dementia, and their carers, to cope with the changes that can
occur in the course of the disease, what other actions beyond
those already described in this chapter are useful? The answer is
to support the carers. We will discuss options for carers in detail
in Chapter Four, but there are a number of carer themes that
practitioners should keep in mind as part of a response to their
patient's changing state. Aspects of the carer role that need
recognition include:

- skills in caring

- need for support

- stress they may be under

- dangers to health

- feelings about the changing relationship with the
  patient: anger, resentment, love, sadness, feelings of
  loss (which are the same, broadly speaking, as those
  experienced by the patient).

Most carers do much more than can be reasonably expected,
sometimes because they have little choice, but often because they
choose to; but it may not always be right to expect the carer to
care. In the case of relatives or friends acting as carers, the quality
of the prior relationship may matter, with their commitment and
capacity to care potentially affected by past conflicts. Here again
the contact between individuals and their general practitioner or
practice nurse over a long period of time may allow both sides to
understand each other better, and to engage in a dialogue about
needs, possibilities and the limits to care-giving.

This kind of dialogue can be supported by more formal and
structured approaches to assessing the needs of the carer, like the
Carers (Recognition and Services) Act 1995. This gives family

carers who are providing, or intending to provide, a 'substantial amount of care on a regular basis' a statutory right to an assessment of their needs. Potential areas to cover in the carer's assessment include:

- their views of the situation

- the nature of their relationship with the cared-for person

- the tasks undertaken and their impact, and the need for help

- their social contacts and the support received from family friends and neighbours

- their emotional, mental and physical health

- their willingness and/or ability to continue to provide care

- options available to the carer, particularly carers who are in employment

- their understanding of the illness or disability of the cared for person and its likely/possible development

- other responsibilities, e.g. work, education, family/childcare commitments

- carers' strengths and ways of coping

- any particular stress factors or aspects of the caring task which the carer finds particularly difficult.

We will return to these issues in Chapter Four, but before that we need to mention an approach to gaining support and assistance that is distinct from the medical model of 'referral' to other agencies – networking.

Networks of support

The existence of a strong network with key individuals working together can help carers care longer. The often unrelenting physical and emotional demands of caring for someone with dementia require sensitive intervention at the point when most needed, so that carers do not feel isolated or alone. Subject to the qualifications about disclosure of the diagnosis that we discussed in Chapter Two, it is very important to tell the carer and the patient about the way in which the illness affects the self and behaviour, because knowing what to expect will help everyone devise strategies for coping. Getting the timing right, and making the right judgements about how to present ideas and issues, may be difficult but are no different in principle from any other situation where bad news needs thought and consideration. We argue that both the GP and other members of the primary care team have a role in counselling both the carer and the person with dementia, without assuming that this role is more important than that of the local Alzheimer's Society branch, or the clinical psychologist in the memory clinic, or the community psychiatric nurse. From the point of view of those affected, the general practitioner and practice nurse are in the network of the patient and the family, and will need to respond to the need for discussion as part of that network.

Family carers of patients with dementia experience prolonged strain, which may result in precipitate admission of the patient to hospital or other institution as well as contributing to physical and mental ill health in the carer. Primary care workers need to know that

- support groups for dementia are valued by carers but may not be enough to reduce the strain of caring

- respite care provides carers with satisfaction but does not appear to alter their overall well-being

- depression is common in carers, and is associated with behavioural problems and higher dependence in the patient and low income in the household, but not with the severity of the cognitive impairment itself

- acknowledging distress in carers and providing more information about dementia increases their satisfaction with services

- men carers complain less about the burden of caring, but experience it as much as women

- the stress of caring is not necessarily reduced by the institutionalization of the dementia sufferer.

In other words, it is the whole picture that determines the process and outcome of care for both the individual with dementia and those around her. No single, simple solutions are likely to be enough to stabilize worsening situations and enhance the quality of life of anyone concerned, but multiple responses may help.

Support and information

One useful action that can be taken by any nurse or doctor with a patient with dementia is to offer sources of useful information. The Alzheimer's Society provides information about all major causes of dementia, and support for families with an individual with dementia through its 300 branches in England, Wales and Northern Ireland. Alzheimer Scotland provides a similar service. As a minimum information package we suggest the following four headings: the details of the support organizations; information about driving, where necessary; pointers about financial issue, which the individuals concerned can discuss in detail with social services, the Citizens Advice Bureau or Alzheimer's Society itself; and an introduction to the legal issues.

Support organisations

The Alzheimer's Society is at Gordon House, 10 Greencoat Place, London SW1P 1PH (tel: 020 7306 0606; email: *info@alzheimers.org.uk*; website: *www.alzheimers.org.uk*). The Alzheimer's Society has services and resources are here to help professionals, as well as people with dementia and their carers:

- a national helpline (0845 300 0336), with a team of advisers available to answer questions on all aspects of dementia, including treatment, care and support

- 300 groups and contacts across the country, offering services and advice at a local level

- grants for carers

- 100 publications, including leaflets, information and advice sheets, reading lists, training resources.

Alzheimer Scotland is based at 22 Drumheugh Gardens, Edinburgh EH3 7RN (tel: 0131 243 1453; fax: 0131 243 1450; email: *alzheimers@alzscot.org;* website: *http://www.alzscot. org/contact.html*. For information or emotional support on any issue to do with dementia call the Scottish 24-hour Dementia Helpline: 0808 808 3000.

Dementia Relief Trust is at 6 Camden High Street London NW1 0JH; tel: 020 7874 7210; fax: 020 7874 7219; email: *info@dementiarelief.org.uk*; website: *http://www. dementiarelief.org .uk/index.htm*). A national charity providing support for carers of people with dementia, the Dementia Relief Trust was established in 1995 to provide a professional framework for the Admiral Nurse Service, a specialist nursing intervention focused on meeting the needs of carers of people with dementia. The organization has a remit to: promote and develop new Admiral Nurse teams; support and sustain existing Admiral Nurse

services; and provide high-quality training for professionals
working with older people, carers and people with dementia.

Driving

The patient has a legal duty to inform the DVLA if diagnosed as
having dementia. They may be given a Group 1 licence, if there is
no significant deterioration in time and space awareness, and
retention of insight and judgement, but an annual medical
review is needed for renewal. The GP should inform the DVLA if
the patient cannot understand this advice

Legal issues

Family carers should be encouraged to seek advice and background information from the Alzheimer's Society on enduring
power of attorney, the Court of Protection and the Public Trust
Office, and guardianship.

To sum up, in this chapter we have reviewed the issues about
the experience of dementia, from the viewpoint of the patient
and those around them, outlined the problems that may challenge carers and primary care professionals, placed medication
use in context and alerted the reader to carers' issues. In the next
chapters we will consider the caring role in more detail, explore
team-working further, and finally summarize some aspects of
good practice in clinical care and in the commissioning services
for dementia.

CHAPTER FOUR

Carers of People with Dementia

> It's now six months since 5.3 million people watched *Malcolm and Barbara ... a love story* (a televised BBC documentary of the daily life of Malcolm and Barbara Pointon) ... Then the personal letters and phone calls started to arrive – literally hundreds of them and so many saying, 'Your story is my story'. Reading some of these highly personal accounts and feeling the loving sympathy with which they were written often reduced me to tears. Thank you ... Interestingly, some letters came from GPs and health professionals. Several said they had no idea life could be so tough for the family carer. (Barbara Pointon, carer of Malcolm Pointon, writing in the Alzheimer's Society Newsletter, p. 4, January 2000)

Barbara Pointon is one of the estimated 5.7 million informal carers in the UK (Office for National Statistics 1998). She provides anecdotal evidence of the self-confessed lack of knowledge that health professionals have about the experience of caring for someone with dementia. In this chapter we offer an overview of this caring experience and signpost sources of further information. We also use suggestion strategies which can be employed by primary health care professionals to assist carers in their particular and highly personal pathway of caring.

FAMILIES, DEMENTIA AND CARING

Most people who develop dementia have a kinship network. Kin and the other people close to the person with dementia are affected in a multitude of ways by the progress of this chronic disease. The roles, responsibilities and expectations of the close family change with the progress of the dementia. The feelings and problems that result all interact, making it a powerful and painful experience for all. Anyone working with families of people with dementia needs to be aware of this.

The greater part of care for people with dementia is provided by their relatives. Invariably, attention focuses on the primary care giver, the significant other person, usually sharing a home, upon whom the person with dementia comes increasingly to rely for the achievement of all their everyday activities. National data on primary carers is available from the General Household Survey (Office for National Statistics 1998) and from this data we know that people who provide care are

- more likely to be women than men

- more likely to be between 45 and 64 than any other age group

- more likely to be a relative than not

- more likely to be looking after someone aged over 75

- more likely than not to be the spouse (equal number of men and women), if the dependent person is elderly and married.

We do not know much more about those who care for people with dementia, a situation that may be remedied by the new question on caring in the 2001 census (Department of Health 2000). There is some evidence that there are large numbers of people who have secondary caring roles. Estimates in the early 1990s suggested a population of 320,000 people with advanced cognitive impairment. Of these 60 per cent (i.e about 192,000) would be living at home and of these 80 per cent (i.e. about 153,600) would be living with informal carers (Schneider *et al.* 1993). However this type of statistics can never capture two points which need to be remembered by the primary care professional. These are that

- to focus on the primary care giver is to ignore that there are often others (usually family members) who form a network of relationships in the caring process and who may be profoundly affected by the progress of the dementia

- the role of carer mirrors the changes in the progress of the dementia; this role changes and continues, even if the person with dementia is living in an institutional setting.

THE ROLE OF CARER AND CARING

The pathway of care giving reflects the pathway of the dementia and has major points of transition. Therefore care-giving and being a care giver are dynamic activities and states, although there may be long periods in the pathway of care where little change appears to happen. Many commentators have described this carer pathway as a 'career'. Aneshenshel identified three career stages which for primary health care practitioners with long-term relationships with care givers can usefully understand (Aneshensel *et al.* 1995). These stages are:

- *role acquisition* – including recognition and preparation for the care giver role

- *role enactment* – enactment of care-related tasks and responsibilities within the home and possibly institutional care

- *role disengagement* – the changes following cessation of care-giving following the death of the person with dementia.

These stages match the stages of reaction and adjustment that individuals with dementia experience, as described at the beginning of Chapter Three. The onset of family care-giving is often not distinguishable from the mutual exchange of assistance. This gradual onset means that initially the care giver does not recognize or label themselves as a 'carer' and may not have made any conscious decisions about assuming this role. Assuming a greater care-giving role is predicated on a range of motivations such as affection, kinship, obligation, reciprocity, lack of quality alternatives (Clarke 1999) and situational factors such as geography.

The notions of *career* and *transition* are very helpful in understanding change in roles and relationships. All care givers start off in one role, such as husband or daughter, with a history and way of being in their personal relationships with this other adult. As the dementia progresses, parts of this original role recede and the care giver assumes some or all of the following roles:

- *decision maker* – with, and then on behalf of, the person

- *protector* – preserving the self-image of the person, as well as physically protecting from harm

- *advocate* – promoting the interests of the person with dementia

- *supervisor* – ensuring the person with dementia is able to undertake activities appropriately

- *monitor* – observing changes in the individual as well as the quality of care provided by others

- *instrumental carer* – providing the activities of daily living, including the physical, emotional and social tasks the person with dementia can no longer perform

- *preserver* – repository of knowledge about the person who can no longer communicate for themselves their history, their personality or their preferences.

It is important to understand this range of roles and that they change over time. Separating them out this way also helps elucidate how others in the care-giving network can contribute even when they are not providing direct physical care. However, this is not to underestimate that different members within a family network can hold completely different beliefs and motivations about care-giving. Primary health care professionals will recognize from experience how a family network can as easily generate conflict as concordance in caring. The following case study illustrates this.

CASE STUDY 6

Mr R began to develop symptoms of dementia in his mid-sixties. He shared a flat with his daughter Elizabeth, 20 years younger than himself, who worked full-time. His wife had died when their daughter was five. His son Michael lived 200 miles away and had a young family. Mr R's brother and family lived in a different part of the same city but had never been close. The dementia progressed over a period of years during which Elizabeth, with support from a network of neighbours and use of a day centre, helped Mr R maintain his independence at home. Mr R's brother visited two or three times a year but never became a regular part of the care network. However, there came a point when the daughter could no longer cope with the aggressive behaviour, incontinence, broken sleep

---

patterns and repeated attempts to 'go home' (to his childhood home) culminating in becoming lost one night and being found by the police. Elizabeth and Michael agreed, after much painful discussion, that the way forward was to seek residential care. Mr R was admitted to an assessment in-patient unit. At this point Mr R's brother visited Elizabeth and a furious row ensued. He argued that it was her duty to look after her father at home, that he was appalled that a member of his family should end up in care being looked after by strangers and that this would give the wrong sort of impression to neighbours, friends and members of his church. Professionals working with Mr R found themselves repeatedly petitioned by his brother to support his views. Elizabeth was so outraged at her uncle's attitudes and lack of practical help that she refused ever to speak to him or his family again. She kept to her word during the remaining 12 months of Mr R's life and at his funeral.

The case study highlights potentially difficult relationships between professionals and members of the family and caring network. A number of commentators have pointed out the ambiguous nature of the relationships between family carers with professionals, in the sense that family carers can be perceived either as a problem in their own right or as a solution to another person's problems (Twigg 1989). This ambiguity requires primary care professionals to consider which view of carers they use in their work (Twigg and Atkin 1994). If we analyse potential perspectives on carers we can identify the following and must then consider which are the most applicable in any given situation. The carer may be

- a resource to deal with the problems of the person with dementia

- a co-client/patient to the person with dementia
- a co-worker with the professionals
- an active co-producer of their own well-being.

THE IMPACT OF CARING FOR SOMEONE WITH DEMENTIA

As we have tried to outline above, being a carer is not a static or homogeneous state. It is important to point out that there are positive aspects to being a carer before we look at the more negative consequences, if only because health and social care professionals rarely think about the positive aspects (Grant and Nolan 1993). Carers of people with dementia have described satisfaction in caring stemming from: a feeling of job satisfaction; a way of expressing ongoing affection and love; continued reciprocity; companionship; and the fulfilment of a sense of duty (Murray *et al.* 1999). However, there is an increasing body of knowledge which demonstrates how this role has negative effects on carers' lives, particularly primary carers. The impact can be described in four interacting domains – economic, social, mental and physical – although these domains may be experienced differently by individual care givers. We will look at these domains in turn and identify relevant initiatives for primary care teams to consider.

Economic impact

The economic impact on carers includes:

- the costs incurred while caring
- reduction of income through giving up paid work for some carers
- reduction of future financial security and pension for some carers

(Caring Costs Alliance 1996)

Carers as a group tend to experience lower income levels than non-carers. Female sole carers who are co-resident with the person with dementia experience the greatest financial disadvantage (Victor 1997). A postal survey of 2000 members of the Carers National Association (Holzhausen and Pearlman 2000) reported that three-quarters stated their financial position was worse since becoming a carer; a third had no savings; a third reported they had trouble paying their utility bills; 60 per cent reported that their financial worries affected their health. In a study of 78 adult carers of parents with dementia, depression was significantly associated with a lower income (Dura *et al.* 1991). It has been demonstrated repeatedly that primary health care is an excellent venue from which to offer financial advice and improve state benefit take up. There are increasing examples where, through collaborative initiatives with general practice and community health services, welfare rights officers have increased the income of older people (Iliffe and Lenihan 2000).

At a minimum, members of the primary health care team should be conversant with and ready to pass on to carers, the relevant main state benefits and local sources of advice regarding these. The relevant state benefits are:

- invalid care allowance for carers

- attendance allowance for people aged over 65

- disability living allowance care component for people aged under 65

- reduction in or exemption from council tax.

The Benefits Agency provides an information service through the national Benefits Enquiry Line (0800 882 200).

Social impact

The impact on the social life of carers includes the effect on their interpersonal relationships with others through increased levels of social isolation. Increasing social isolation is common. Carers who live with a person with dementia report how friends lose contact as the dementia progresses, and attribute this to a range of causes including the friends' inability to cope with the changes, or the seeming inappropriateness of invitations for social events for someone with dementia. One study of 176 carers, which compared male and female carers of people with dementia, showed that the male carers tended to withdraw from their social network when taking over the caring role. The stigma that is still associated with 'senility' and 'mental health problems' should not be underestimated. All too many carers and people with dementia find that previously friendly and approachable people become embarrassed and strained in their presence.

In practical terms, the ability of the carer to continue to participate in social activities is dependent on the availability of others to keep company with the person with dementia. Forty-five per cent of carers surveyed in 1998 reported they received no help with the person they cared for (Carers National Association 1996). The link between being able to maintain a social life and emotional well-being is very important for carers of people with dementia. Feelings of loneliness and of having no time for leisure activities are implicated in the high levels of poor psychological health reported by carers of people with dementia (Buck, Gregson and Bamford 1997). We need now to turn to these other domains to explore the impact on the care giver.

Mental and physical impact

The emotional, mental and physical impact of caring includes increased experience of stress and distress, increased rates of depression, prolonged bereavement, and physical injury through caring (e.g. back injuries).

> I love my husband dearly but because he has Alzheimer's disease he is no god. I am so stressed that I scream and say the most hurtful things to him and then hate myself afterwards.
> (RL, Essex, Alzheimer's Society Newsletter, June 1997)

There is an increasing body of evidence pointing to the physical and psychological impact of caring for another person. A recent cross sectional survey of 4550 adults in England identified that prevalence of psychiatric morbidity was significantly higher in the 10 per cent of respondents who cared for others in their own homes (Horsley *et al.* 1998). A postal survey of 5000 carers revealed that 51 per cent of carers had suffered a physical injury such as back strain and 52 per cent reported themselves as having been treated for stress-related illnesses since they began to care (Henwood 1998).

Caring for someone with a deteriorating condition such as dementia is characterized by stress and distress, affecting physical and emotional well-being. Anyone caring for people with dementia knows this to be the reality, and the studies only confirm their experience. A high incidence of chronic fatigue, depression and other psychological problems has been demonstrated in carers of people with dementia in numerous studies since the early 1980s. An increased incidence of depression is associated with behavioural problems and with situations where higher levels of care are required by the person with dementia (Russo and Vitaliano 1995). For some carers the levels of stress and distress can become unbearable as hinted at in this anonymous reader's letter:

> I have long been sickened rather than inspired by the testimony of apparently selfless, loving carers. I believe that Mrs B (a previous letter writer) and I are part of a silent majority: resentful, longing for release from a hateful burden

while knowing that release will come too late to appreciate it.
(Alzheimer's Society Newsletter, June 1997)

However, what is not clear in the many studies of the
psychological impact of caring for people with dementia is the
interplay between grief, stress and depression. In common with
carers of other people with degenerative impairments, carers of
people with dementia experience multiple bereavements over the
course of the illness. They lose not only elements of the person
with dementia but also parts of their own life and future
expectations. Carers of people with dementia experience
repeated grieving with all that it entails – denial, acute and
episodic pangs of grief, anger, resentment, guilt, sadness and
adaptation. At each significant event in the course of the
dementia the carer grieves, begins to accept the change, begins
to adapt, only to encounter another loss, triggering a further
round of grief.

> Mum gently slept away to peace in my arms after 8 years in
> care. I felt a sense of relief that she had been released from
> this dreadful disease. Relief too for myself. I am coping
> surprisingly well and without trying those last ten years seem
> to have been put away in a special box in my memory. When I
> think of Mum now the happy days come back and I take this
> as my inspiration. I have already grieved for ten years. (KD,
> Goole, Alzheimer's Society Newsletter, February 1999)

So how can primary care professionals help, carers with the
sometimes overwhelming impact of caring for people with
dementia? Interestingly, after decades of describing the
problems, little is known about the effectiveness of interventions
to address or ameliorate them. A recent systematic review
underlined the paucity of high-quality research in this area of
practice (Thompson and Thompson 1998). Research studies
using randomized control trials on interventions such as a)
referral to groups for the provision of support and information;
b) regular respite services; c) carer training; and d) multi-

dimensional assessment and support have not shown significant statistical impact on carers' mental well-being. However, without fail, these are the sorts of services and actions that carers repeatedly request, often retrospectively, or praise if they gain access to them. It would seem important to look at what carers themselves say they need to help them.

CARERS' VIEWS

Throughout the 1990s there were studies, surveys and carers' projects which collated carers' views on what help they need and how they want to be treated (see, for example, Bamford *et al.* 1998). These identify key principles which carers report as necessary for a good quality of life for the person they care for, and for themselves. These principles are now incorporated in the first government National Strategy for Carers (Department of Health 2000) outlined below. Carers want:

- full information on all issues pertinent to the quality of their life and of the cared for person's life

- recognition as carers and acknowledgement of their own health needs, including emotional support

- reliable, high-quality services for the person they care for and for themselves

- time for their own life – whether that's maintaining paid employment or with friends and family – through planned breaks in caring

- training, advice and support to care

- financial security

- inclusion by professionals of their contribution and knowledge in both their individual situation and the review and development of local services.

My wife was diagnosed with Alzheimer's 10 years ago. Our GP (whom we have known for 30 years) recognised her symptoms immediately as his own mother had the same illness for 9 years. Sending my wife for scans etc. confirmed his diagnosis. But he never once told me what to expect, how the disease would develop, how far ahead we should look. He said there was nothing we could do. But if he had only taken the time to show me, teach me how to handle the situation, perhaps we would have made better use of the time when she could still talk and walk. (CM, Woodford Green, Alzheimer's Society Newsletter, April 1999)

The availability of statutory service provision to help carers take breaks from caring is a geographical lottery in the UK (Fruin 1998). Those carers who do have access to services to help them take a break – whether day care, sitting services or relief care – reported that it had improved the quality of their lives at that point. Primary care professionals can assist carers by making sure they have the information on accessing local carer networks and services that provide carers with break at an early point in their caring career, rather than when crisis develops.

Wherever we met carers in touch with carers' groups or carers' centres we heard almost nothing but praise for how these provided sensitive emotional support as well as serving as effective sources of information for carers about services and procedures and in some cases direct services. (Fruin 1998, section 1.19)

RESPONDING TO CHALLENGES?

The National Carers Strategy offers a policy framework focused for the first time on the needs of carers. Its main elements are based on

- improving information to carers

- improving support to carers (including financial) – reinforcing their right under legislation to have an assessment of their needs

- improving the provision of care to carers and care break facilities. In doing this it sets out some good practice principles in the form of questions for GPs and primary health care teams which are reproduced in Box 4.1.

BOX 4.1 CHECKLIST FOR GPS AND PRIMARY CARE TEAMS TO HELP CARERS

- Have you identified those of your patients who are carers, and patients who have a carer? Do you check carers' physical and emotional health whenever a suitable opportunity arises, and at least once a year?

- Do you routinely tell carers that they can ask social services for an assessment of their own needs?

- Do you always ask patients who have carers whether they are happy for health information about them to be told to their carer?

- Do you know whether there is a carers' support group or carers' centre in your area, and do you tell carers about them?

(Department of Health 2000, p.57)

This checklist could easily form the starting point for a practice team or multidisciplinary group to enhance their service for patients with dementia and their carers, either by providing standards for a baseline assessment of their work or by identifying which systems, processes and information they need. The checklist has been expanded below to be more specific to carers of people with dementia, and we commend it to practitioners as a tool for improving service quality.

Checklist for primary care professionals on working with carers of people with dementia

- Do you know who is a carer of a person with dementia?

- Is the fact that they are a carer easily identifiable on records available to all members of the team?

- Do you have a system for ensuring that each carer is given *written* information on

  - sources of information on dementia, dementia management, caring for people with dementia

  - state benefits associated with caring

  - Alzheimer's Society address and telephone number (particularly local branches)

  - local carers' services/centres with address and telephone number

  - Carers National and Alzheimer's Society helpline numbers

  - their right to have their needs assessed under the Carers (Recognition and Services) Act 1995 by social services and the local system for that assessment

  - local training and learning initiatives for carers of people with dementia

  - local availability and system for providing breaks for carers?

- Do you have a system of proactively identifying change in both the carers' health status and their need for support in caring? (And does this specifically address the high incidence of depression?)

- Is there information available to the team detailing the local services (specialist or otherwise) that can assist carers of people with dementia and how to refer to them?

- Have your team identified a way of supporting carers experiencing acute episodes of bereavement?

My family has in the past suffered at the hands of GPs who do not have the time or inclination to support carers. At last I can honestly praise the actions of my mother's present GP. We had yet another stage of this harrowing disease thrust upon us. Repeated infections and poor swallowing reflexes resulted in invasive antibiotic injections, suction pumps and even a mention of intravenous feeding. It was the GP who suggested a family meeting to discuss the current problems and how we might deal with them. He had obviously put a great deal of thought into the situation and showed empathy and compassion. He couldn't take away the pain or guilt but I came away wanting to wrap him up and distribute him nation wide. (JD, Fenay Bridge, Alzheimer's Society Newsletter, February 1999)

**BOX 4.2 A SOURCE OF INFORMATION
FOR CARERS AND FAMILIES**

Mace, N.L., Rabins, P.V. et al. (1992) The 36 Hour Day: *A Family Guide to Caring at Home for People with Alzheimer's Disease and Other Confusional Illnesses* (2nd edition) London: Hodder & Stoughton and Age Concern.

CHAPTER FIVE

Caring for People as the Dementia Progresses

> My mother died last year, nine years after the onset of dementia. She lived at home with my father for five years, then they moved near to me, where she lived with him for another two years. After they moved, several very kind carers and I provided some help. When my father reached a point when he could no longer continue caring for her full time, I decided for many reasons not to do it myself. Having explored the limited alternatives, we took the agonising decision to opt for full time residential care in one of only two nursing homes in our area with a special dementia unit. (Finch 2000, p.14)

In this chapter we consider issues that arise when supporting people with dementia and their carers as the dementia progresses beyond the early losses. The progress and extent of the dementia is different for each person. It has been eloquently argued that the pathway cannot be understood purely from a standpoint of neuropathology but that each person's personality, biography, physical health and social psychology are also important (Kitwood 1997). A person with dementia experiences multiple changes, including:

- progressive failure of mental powers such as memory, reasoning and comprehension

- loss of social interaction skills

- loss of psycho-motor skills.

This progression can mean that the person loses a range of abilities as illustrated in Table 5.1. However, we know that the experience of dementia is influenced by the availability or absence of support and services, and in particular the extent to which the person with dementia is enabled to use their abilities and interact with others. To describe the progress of dementia in neat progressive 'stages' ignores these other influences and channels formal and informal carers into creating care environments which provide self-fulfilling prophecies (Bell and McGregor 1995). In other words, if individuals are not encouraged to use their memory skills, they will not appear to have any.

Table 5.1 Outline of the effect of progressing dementia		
Domain within the person	Potential progression of dementia → → → → →	
Memory	May not recognize familiar people and places	Poor recent and distant memory of people, places, events
	May not remember to undertake activities of their daily life such as eating or taking drinks	see **Self-maintenance** domain below
Cognition and comprehension	Difficulty in making decisions and plans	Loss of cognitive abilities
	Difficulty in comprehending the written word, writing and making calculations	
	Difficulty in comprehending others' actions, speech and how others feel	Loss of comprehension of speech, interpreting others' actions or feelings
	Unable to judge own physical appearance	

Communication	Speech becoming slower and impoverished, repetition of certain words and phrases	Inability to communicate with words but may use word fragments, single words, shouts and cries
Emotions	Emotionally labile, and may develop strong emotional reactions to seemingly minor events	Display emotions often in non-verbal ways
Physical	May develop repetitive physical patterns, such as a need to keep walking or wiping surfaces	
	Walking may become more problematic, and they are more likely to bump into things or fall	Inability to walk or move large muscles
	Difficulties with perceptual motor co-ordination, e.g. sitting down in the right place on a chair	
Self-maintenance	Gradual loss of ability to wash, dress or feed themselves without assistance	Inability to maintain themselves physically without assistance
Continence	May experience incontinence through inability to recognize stimuli or comprehend an appropriate place to void	Inability to control bladder and bowel functions

Among others the late Tom Kitwood, a clinical psychologist, explored these issues in depth (Kitwood and Bredin 1992). He argued that reliance on a neuropathological framework for understanding the progress of dementia, combined with a history of dehumanizing institutional care traditions, has supported a 'malignant social psychology' in caring for people with dementia. This malignant social psychology in professionals and carers, while not intentionally evil, reduces the person to an object and fails to recognize the importance to them of the psychosocial environment. Kitwood and his colleagues have listed 17 methods which formal and informal carers use to take away the status of 'person' from someone with dementia. Their ideas derive in the main from observations in institutional settings. These depersonalizing techniques are compounded by a form of neglect – the absence of provision of human interaction and occupation for long periods of time. The extent to which primary care professionals participate in or create such a malignant psychology has not been explored. In Box 5.1 we have given some examples of ways in which the status of 'person' can be undermined. We invite you use this list to consider how you and your own colleagues work with someone with dementia.

BOX 5.1 METHODS INVOLVED IN REMOVING THE STATUS OF PERSON FROM SOMEONE WITH DEMENTIA (adapted from Kitwood 1997, pp.46–47)

1. *Treachery* – forms of deception to manipulate the person or gain compliance; e.g. saying that the visit to the hospital is just for a few tests when in fact the person is being taken to a new residential home

2. *Disempowerment* – not allowing the person to use the abilities they do have, failing to help them complete actions they have initiated; e.g. advising the carer on how to feed the person because it is quicker and less messy than letting them do it themselves

3. *Infantilization* – treating them as an insensitive parent might treat a very young child; e.g. public, loud chastisement after an episode of incontinence

4. *Intimidation* – inducing fear in a person through threats; e.g. making threats that the person will have to go into a residential home if they don't stop getting up in the middle of the night and turning all the lights on

5. *Labelling* – using the category of dementia as the main basis for interacting with the person or to

---

explain their behaviour; e.g saying that people with dementia always experience distress rather than looking for explanations particular to that person such as the death of someone close

6. *Stigmatization* – treating a person as if they were an alien or an outcast; e.g. hostile comments/looks from receptionists and others in waiting rooms as the person with dementia waiting for a long time becomes more agitated, pacing around

7. *Outpacing* – providing information, presenting choices at a rate too fast for the person to understand; e.g. telling someone about the clinical procedure you are about to do at the same moment as you start doing it

8. *Invalidation* – failing to acknowledge the subjective reality of a person's experience and especially what they are feeling; e.g. only asking for information from a carer in a consultation with a person with dementia even though they are sitting side by side

9. *Banishment* – sending a person away, or excluding them, e.g. always leaving a person with dementia to sit alone in the front room with the TV on while the rest of the family congregate and carry on domestic life in another room

10. *Objectification* – treating the person as if they were an inert thing, to be pushed, moved or filled without reference to the fact they are sentient beings; e.g. physically washing and dressing someone without talking to them or acknowledging any of their actions or reactions

FOCUSING ON THE PERSON

Over the last ten years much has been done to increase awareness of the ways in which care becomes depersonalized and fails to address the social-psychological needs of the person with dementia. This work includes:

- education and awareness raising for professionals

- recognizing the views and perceptions of people with dementia

- appropriate frameworks for assessment, including risk, and care planning for people with dementia

- specific evaluation of care to people with dementia.

Education and awareness raising

We discuss multidisciplinary educational initiatives applied to primary health care in Chapter Six. It is also important to note that as in all attempts to change attitudes and professional practice, the wider context of barriers to change have to be addressed (Lintern, Woods and Phair 2000). The wider context of personal and organizational barriers are important to address and plan for through change management techniques (Dawson 1992).

The views of people with dementia

Recognition of the status of 'person' means that the views and participation of the person with dementia in assessment, care planning and monitoring are integral. The challenge in working with people who have dementia is of course that communication can be compromised by a breakdown in language processing, a breakdown in motor speech production or a breakdown in other cognitive processes. Studies and practical work over the last ten years have shown that clear and creative strategies are necessary to help communication take place with and for people with dementia (Goldsmith 1996). Some of the more creative techniques have included life story work, reminiscence work, prose and poetry creation. Practical communication skills are essential for primary care professionals in working with the person with dementia. We give some suggestions below and provide information in Box 5.2 on further reading for helping to hear the voice of people with dementia.

The following are suggestions in practical communication skills:

- Reduce the chance of alarming the person by approaching them in their line of vision, and conduct your conversation at a similar voice level to theirs.

- Ensure the surrounding environment does not provide competing distractions.

- Make sure all aids to communication are operational, e.g. glasses in place, hearing aids switched on.

- Reinforce your words with non-verbal communication, i.e. try to make and keep eye contact; use a calm, reassuring tone; consider using touch, such as holding hands if appropriate; illustrate your words with pictures or the real thing, e.g. the stethoscope.

- Be a good listener and observer of non-verbal clues. Remember that the person with dementia may use 'concrete symbols' instead of abstract concepts like feelings.

- Allow enough time between statements and actions for comprehension and responses.

- Use short, jargon-free, simple sentences which deal with one issue at a time.

- Avoid complicated linguistic devices, such as rhetorical questions and the royal 'we'.

BOX 5.2 FURTHER READING: HEARING THE VOICE OF PEOPLE WITH DEMENTIA

Crisp, J. (2000) *Keeping in Touch with Someone Who Has Alzheimer's.* AusMed Publications, Australia

Goldsmith, M. (1996) *Hearing the Voice of People with Dementia.* Jessica Kingsley, London

Killick, J. (2000) *Openings: Dementia Poems and Photographs.* Hawker Publications, London

Murphy, C. and Moyes, M. (1997) 'Life Story Work.' In M. Marshall (ed) *State of the Art in Dementia Care.* Centre for Policy on Ageing, London

---

However, do not underestimate the practical negotiating skills required in situations where the person with dementia may be very apprehensive and has relied on high levels of collusion by others to minimize their problems.

> Robert (the professional assessor) had a very careful, casual approach. There were no forms at all. My husband was worried at first. He doesn't know anything is wrong with him but Robert made the effort to gain his trust. Robert kept chatting. He avoided asking direct questions – it was a deliberate ploy. (Quote from an interview with a carer given in Moriarty and Webb 2000, p.40)

One other development that will be of value to primary care professionals is the establishment of advocacy schemes for people with dementia, mooted first in the mid-1980s (Kings Fund 1986). These are usually based on models of citizens' advocacy 'where a trained volunteer develops a relationship with their partner (or client) and stands alongside them in speaking up for their rights. Their role is to work out with their partner what they want and to make representations to necessary agencies in order to gain this' (Goodchild 1999, p.619). The majority of these schemes tend to be focused on residential settings, but there is clearly scope for their development for people who remain in their own homes.

Appropriate systems of assessment, care planning and monitoring

As the dementia progresses, the person with dementia and their carers require greater levels of assistance – either at home or in some form of care setting. Primary health care professionals have to have knowledge and systems to offer their own expertise at the right points while helping the person with dementia and carers access those other services they need.

> The nature of dementia is of an ever-changing downward spiral and it is very hard to predict accurately when the wheels of support should be put in motion. But believe me when we need help we need it *now*! The formal part of the proceedings could be started soon after diagnosis even though it may be months – or years – until help is actually sought … Assessment, form-filling and locating required documentation takes months and only exacerbates our stress when in crisis. (Nurock 2000, p.27)

One of the great organizational challenges in this is how to reduce the number of times the person with dementia and their carer have to answer the same questions in the assessment processes of different professionals. Sharing records, two or more professionals meeting with the person with dementia and their carers at the same time – these are just two of the ideas that could be tested more widely.

Access to a greater level of assistance for the majority of people is achieved through the community care assessment process led by a Social Services Care Manager. In some areas a care programme approach through mental health services is used with people whose dementia has severely incapacitated them

(Social Services Inspectorate 1996). Local differences in procedures, in charging systems for care and in responsibilities between health and social services for long-term care, make it important for primary care professionals to understand (and share this understanding with carers) the local system they contribute to. The checklist in Box 5.3 can be used to identify gaps in primary health care professionals' local knowledge of the community care assessment processes. Try it on yourself.

BOX 5.3 A CHECKLIST OF KNOWLEDGE OF THE LOCAL COMMUNITY CARE ASSESSMENT PROCESSES

- Do you know what the published local authority eligibility criteria for simple and complex community care assessments are?

- Do you know how to make a referral for a complex community care assessment and advise carers how to get an assessment of their own needs under the Carers Recognition Act?

- Do you know how your assessment and care planning processes fit with those undertaken by care managers from the social services departments?

- Do you know what the local social service department policy on charging for services is and what their upper financial limit is for supporting an individual in their own home?

- Do you know what the local system is for agreeing whether a person with dementia is the financial responsibility of the NHS or the local authority in meeting their long-term continuing health or community care needs?

There are no standardized assessment and care planning documents in use across health and social services (Moriarty and

Webb 2000). However, there are some, such as CarenapD (Cameron and Chapman 2000), which have been developed specifically to direct a multiprofessional group to consider the strengths, preferences and needs of the person with dementia. CarenapD provides the following prompts as to the types of help the person with dementia might need:

- social stimulation/activity – where someone provides company and/or activities

- prompting/supervision – where someone is there to ensure the person manages, through verbal or physical prompts

- physical assistance – where a helper does the tasks for the person

- aids and adaptations – either for the person or the environment

- specialist assessment – where more detailed expertise is required, for example from an occupational therapist

- counselling for the person – to assist with emotional coping

- behaviour management – strategies to address, cope with and/or diminish behaviour issues

- carer advice/training – to help informal and formal carers help the person.

Risk, rights and responsibilities

One issue which provokes considerable anxiety is the perception and understanding of 'risk' for the person with dementia.

Some tensions were reported between some Social Service Department (SSD) and health staff because of the lack of common understanding about what constituted reasonable risk taking, health personnel sometimes perceiving SSD staff as tending to focus too strongly on the civil liberties of service users. (Social Services Inspectorate 1997, section 8.4)

Risk is perceived differently by different individuals. Balancing risks with the rights and abilities of the individual needs more than one perspective as well as careful individualized assessment and planning. Concerns about things which *might* happen to the person need to be evaluated in terms of possibility, imminence and gravity, and to be balanced against the actual evidence of the particular concerns occurring (Baragwanath 1997). Joint working in assessing risk and using creative as well as technological strategies to reduce risk are imperative. The case study of Margaret G in Chapter Three shows how such joint working can solve difficult problems, over time, with input from a range of different professionals. Box 5.4 provides some suggestions of further reading related to practical issues in assessing and managing risk for people with dementia.

5.4 FURTHER READING: ASSESSING AND MANAGING RISK FOR PEOPLE WITH DEMENTIA

Alzheimer's Society (1994) *Safe as Houses: Living Alone with Dementia.* A resource book to aid risk management. Alzheimer's Society, London

Alzheimer's Society (2000) *Living Alone.* Advice sheet. Alzheimer's Society, London

Marshall, M. (2000) ASTRID: *A Guide to Using Technology Within Dementia Care.* Hawker Publications, London

---

The following case study for you to consider is not resolved in the same way as the case of Margaret G in Chapter Three. How would you try to solve the problem described?

CASE STUDY 7

Mrs L is in her late eighties and has been diagnosed with dementia. She lives alone in her poorly maintained ground floor flat. She has one daughter who lives at a distance. Her condition has recently deteriorated significantly. She had been supported by home care services in maintaining her personal hygiene and nutrition for some time but has increasingly refused to let them help. Problems with lights fusing has meant she has started to use candles for light rather than electricity. She has also started emptying her night commode from her bedroom window next to the front door, much to the concern of her upstairs neighbours. The neighbours have contacted the environmental health department, the social services department as well as the GP, the practice nurse and the practice receptionists. On one occasion in this period Mrs L was returned home in the middle of the night by the police who found her waiting for the supermarket to open. Mrs L has refused any other help when approached by the social worker. She is clear that she wants to stay in her own home of 30 years. Her daughter supports her mother's wishes as she feels that any changes to her accommodation could make her mother's condition worse. The social work care manager finds herself in a difficult position in seeing a way forward as the different parties concerned take increasingly entrenched positions on what the level of risk is.

Evaluating quality of care for people with dementia

So how do primary health care professionals assess the quality of care they provide for people with dementia? Health and social care professionals are notorious for assessing, planning, giving care and then omitting to evaluate, monitor or review the actions at a subsequent point. When we do review or monitor the care plan and the person, what indicators do we use for *well-being* in the person with dementia? Kitwood argues that health and social care professionals do not pay enough attention to how the individual's psychological needs are addressed – specifically the need for comfort, for emotional attachment, for social inclusion, and for occupation (Kitwood 1997). He, with others, has offered ideas for how to gauge well-being in a person with dementia. A simple checklist, devised originally for formal and informal carers to map the well-being of individual people over a period of days, has been developed into the Dementia Care Mapping Method (Bradford Dementia Group 1997) for formal carers working with groups of people with dementia. It uses techniques of observation by staff members 'mapping' the experience and reactions of individual people with dementia and then feeding that back to their colleagues. Table 5.2 is an adaptation of

Table 5.2 Recording of signs of well-being in a person with dementia (adapted from Kitwood and Bredin 1992)

Signs of well-being	Day 1	2	3	4	5	6	7
Being able to assert own will and desires							
Being able to show a range of emotions including pleasure and sadness							
Initiating contact with others							
Having self-respect							
Enjoying humour							
Showing pleasure							
Being able to relax							
Being helpful							
Signs of ill-being							
Distress or despair							
Intense anger							
Physical discomfort/pain							
Fear/anxiety							

Kitwood and Bredin's checklist of signs of well-being in a person with dementia, which could be used as a starting point to consider the well-being of the person with dementia over a period of a week.

We will return to these issues later in the chapter when we discuss issues of inadequate or abusive care as well as in Chapter Six in our discussion of clinical governance.

PRIMARY HEALTH CARE IN RESIDENTIAL AND NURSING HOMES

Much of what we have discussed in this chapter applies as much to people with dementia who live in group settings as it does to individuals still in their homes, or living with family members. Primary care professionals provide care in these settings, and it is issues related to this that we wish to consider.

GPs and nurses are often involved at the point where the decision is made to use a group home as a break, for carers in the home, or as a permanent move into a care residence. Giving up your home or asking someone to leave their home is a major life event for the person with dementia and their relatives. As such it engenders enormous stress and often distress. Primary health care professionals can offer support, opportunities to express emotions and reminders or introductions to the wider local network to share such emotions. Chapter Four outlines issues of carer support as it cannot be forgotten that the carer *remains* a carer when the person with dementia moves to reside in a group setting.

The decision to shift permanent residence is made in different circumstances – sometimes at a point of crisis after emergency admission to hospital – sometimes in a planned, thought-through way. It is a decision invariably associated with factors such as the person with dementia having increased physical dependence, irritability, nocturnal wandering and incontinence, and carer stress (North of England Evidence Based Guidelines

Project 1998). For all concerned it is a move made with a great deal of anxiety and emotion. While primary health care professionals are not likely to have in-depth knowledge to assist in the selection of a residence they need to be able to pass on basic information, such as:

- Social work care managers can supply local lists.

- Registration officers in health authorities and local authorities (shortly to come together) produce both lists and access to published inspection reports.

- There are helpful publications, such as *Home from home: How to Choose a Care Home* (King's Fund, London), and Age Concern's Fact Sheet 29 *Finding Residential and Nursing Home Accommodation*, which lists useful questions to ask when visiting potential homes.

The provision of residential and nursing homes registered for the residence or care of people who are elderly and mentally ill is largely in the independent sector although the finance for an individual's residence may come in full or part from their local authority or health authority. National policy and local interpretation determines issues such as to what extent the public purse supports long-term care of older people, eligibility criteria, and local financial ceilings on the amount for the care of an individual. The question of who should pay for what elements of long-term care for older people is subject to intense political debate at the present time.

Some general practitioners provide medical care for all the residents in a group home, others may have only a small number of patients in a number of homes. Some nursing care is provided by district nurses in residential homes – readers interested in the debate about what constitutes 'nursing' care – the domain of a qualified nurses – and what constitutes 'personal' care – the domain of social care assistants – are directed to the arguments in the report of the Royal Commission on Long Term Care (1999). The reality, however, is that residential homes have increasing numbers of older people who have high levels of physical dependency on others, combined with increased frailty and medical conditions. The increased provision of continence aids and pressure-relieving equipment, such as alternating pressure mattresses in residential homes, via primary care nurses is just one indicator of this (see e.g. Malone and Mackenzie 2000).

> In long term care, as I know from experience, a perceptive doctor can have huge impact on the functioning of the home, the staff and the relatives. It could mean fewer hospital admissions which in themselves are a nightmare. Fewer hospital outpatient appointments with their long waits for transport, a member of staff out for most of the day to accompany them and resulting poorer care for those left behind. (Family carer quoted in Nurock 2000, p.27)

Access to primary health care services is important for people with dementia in residential and nursing homes – not just for immediate health care but also as a gateway to other specialist services. It is also important that relatives are able to access the GP of the person with dementia – particularly if this has changed on entry to a group home. Discussions on emotive issues, such as the level of medical intervention appropriate when a person with dementia becomes seriously ill, for example with pneumonia, are made marginally easier by having prior knowledge of each other, of the relatives' views and of any views the person with dementia may have made known at an earlier time (see Chapter Two). Whatever decision is made, in each situation – based on prior wishes and quality of life – the bottom line for most relatives is that the person with dementia should not experience pain or discomfort, and they look to the GP and nursing staff to use all their palliative care knowledge and skills.

NEGLECT, INADEQUATE CARE AND ABUSE

Before moving on to our final chapter on issues of commissioning, we will touch on one final issue regarding the care experienced by people with dementia in their own home and in group home settings – namely, care that is inadequate, neglectful or abusive. 'Abuse may be described as physical, sexual, psychological or financial. It may be intentional or unintentional or the result of neglect. It causes harm to the older person, either temporarily or over a period of time' (Social Services Inspectorate 1993).

Abuse of older people is not new although it is now more widely recognized. In domestic settings perpetrators can be relatives, friends, volunteers, paid workers and professionals. In institutional settings it can be the act of one person or a reflection of a wider culture where poor standards and poor leadership result in systematic abusive, as well as criminal, acts. A national survey of relatives' experiences of care in residential and nursing homes makes salutary reading (Alzheimer's Society 1997). However, our understanding of how to prevent it remains incomplete. All that we know of the situations and risk factors which make abuse a possibility indicates that people with dementia are extremely vulnerable. A vulnerability compounded by their condition often preventing them from being able to inform others as to what has happened to them or their finances. So what can primary health care professionals do in addressing these complex issues? Here are some suggestions:

- Identify and address your own education needs relating to elder abuse (see Box 5.5 for relevant reading).

- Understand the factors which are likely to increase the risk of abuse and apply this knowledge to all joint assessment and care planning for the person with dementia and their carers.

- Anticipate issues of care stress and help plan to ameliorate them.

- Consider how you would identify the absence of indicators of well-being in your patients with dementia.

- Identify any local guidelines/agreements on action to be taken if abuse is suspected; and if there is none, consider how the principles in national guidance for professionals (Box 5.5) could be applied in your work setting.

- Become more knowledgeable about what high-quality care of people with dementia in groups can be and the standards in the code of good practice for residential and nursing home care (Centre for Policy on Ageing 1996).

- Consider who you would approach, and in what way, if you identified problems in the residential or nursing homes you visited.

BOX 5.5 FURTHER READING: ABUSE OF OLDER PEOPLE

Action on Elder Abuse (1995) *Everybody's Business – Taking Action on Elder Abuse.* Action on Elder Abuse, London

Action on Elder Abuse (1999) *The Abuse of Older People – Information for Doctors.* Action on Elder Abuse, London

Royal College of Nursing (1991) *Guidelines for Nurses: Abuse and Older People.* Royal College of Nursing, London

Slater, P. and Eastman, M. (eds) (1999) *Elder Abuse: Critical Issues in Policy and Practice.* Age Concern England

Social Services Inspectorate (1993) *No Longer Afraid: The Safeguarding of Older People in Domestic Settings.* HMSO, London

Department of Health (2000) *No Secrets. Guidance on Developing Multi-Agency Policies and Procedures to Protect Vulnerable Adults from Abuse.*

CHAPTER SIX

Good Practice and Service Development

The structure of the NHS has changed once again, with fundholding being replaced by primary care groups, which will in turn evolve into larger primary care trusts, or even combined health and social service care trusts. Primary care groups (PCGs), covering populations of about 100,000 people and involving GPs, nurses and social services, are responsible for advising health authorities about commissioning services as well as enhancing the quality of primary care. Primary Care Trusts (PCTs) will both provide services and commission them directly from other providers. Improving the quality of primary care is a major responsibility of PCGs, under the rubric of 'clinical governance', which brings together ideas about standards, evidence-based practice, equity and cost containment. In short, clinical governance will require primary care to provide services that are equitable and just, effective and high quality, and financially prudent. The implications of clinical governance for everyday practice have not yet been grasped by the general practitioners who constitute the majority on PCG management boards, although this may change rapidly. Re-accreditation in general practice is now only a few years away, and professionals with foresight will realise the significance of clinical governance for re-accreditation, and prepare themselves for both. The implications in bringing together systems of quality assurance and financial controls between the health services, the local authorities and the independent sector have scarcely begun to be completed.

How will primary care professionals demonstrate that they are providing optimal care for their patients with dementia, and optimal support to carers? The risk is that demands for information on performance on heart disease prevention or diabetes management will swamp practitioners and practice managers with checklists and quality standards, so that the small number of individuals with dementia will be lost in a bureaucratic paperchase. Similarly, how can professionals from all disciplines enhance their knowledge and skills in dementia care in the community? Learning how to deal with complex and uncommon problems is not easy, but wasting time and resources on ineffective education is simple. Postgraduate teachers will need to think hard about how they approach dementia education, and practitioners will need to reflect on their own practice and its blind-spots.

Finally, how will dementia care fare in this new environment, given the low status given to care for older people in general, and the widespread problems of recognition of and response to dementia in primary care? Will resources flow into counselling and physiotherapy for younger people, perceived as major problems by hard-pressed general practitioners, and away from needier but less vociferous patients whose visibility remains low? How can those working in dementia care prevent adverse selection – the redirection of resources away from those with greatest need – by the new NHS structures?

We have three sets of suggestions to make about these problems, but cannot claim to have all the answers. The route to clinical governance remains unmarked, and all initiatives to provide optimal care in dementia in primary care are exploratory. We offer a template that practitioners can use to assess their own performance, and some hints about information technology and the capture of data. Effective education is better understood, at least in its broad principles, but there is a sizeable educational apparatus with strong leanings towards specialist expertise that needs to be balanced by a more grounded generalist approach. We have suggestions about how to develop an educational programme based on the educational needs of practitioners themselves, not on the needs as seen from the specialist vantage point, not from the ivory tower. And commissioning services is unfamiliar territory for most practitioners of any discipline, in which there are many traps. We describe some of these traps, and ways of avoiding them.

A FRAMEWORK FOR GOOD PRACTICE

We suggest adopting a framework for good practice, which can be applied to all individuals with any form of dementia, whether living in their own home or in a care home. This framework can guide clinical care for individual patients as part of a clinical audit or in a critical incident study, and if used as a template for data capture, can generate the knowledge needed to commission care for a whole population. It has eleven components, which can be reflected in the patient's written or electronic medical record, to optimise case management and also allow audit of the quality of care.

If you have made a diagnosis of dementia check that you have done the following:

1. *Assessed, documented and shared with relevant others the physical, mental, behavioural and social problems of the person with dementia.* For example, the checklist of investigations given in Chapter Two can be used to ensure all baseline tests are done before a diagnosis becomes firm. Similarly, the PAID mnemonic described in Chapter Three can be used to build a template in the record about behaviour problems.

2. *Identified their strengths and remaining skills, and reflected those to them and their family and carers.* This is not so easy to capture, but there may already be a rich history that helps make sense of changes and losses. The previous history of depression may influence decisions about treating depression, and the hobbies and pastimes of the individual with dementia may be important cues for those helping to provide care and support.

3. *Identified what the carer and person with dementia consider to be the main problems and planned a way to address them.* Documenting this may be a challenge, especially in the relatively inflexible medium of electronic records, but achieving it will demonstrate a high degree of patient-centredness.

4. *Identified any treatable complications of coexisting pathology in the patient.* This is a medical task that is, by comparison with the others, easy to perform and record.

5. *Identified the carer's unmet needs and developed a plan to address them.* Here the checklists from Chapter Four may be useful for prompting questions and collating answers.

6. *Provided written information automatically, to at least the carer, on local and national groups and services concerned with dementia.*

7. *Documented levels of assistance and services currently used and identified the appropriate services to meet any unmet needs.* Frameworks such as CaresnapD outlined in Chapter Five are helpful. Is the network of local services understood by all the practitioners, and are the telephone and fax numbers and contact details in the practice and professional's telephone directory?

8. *Reviewed the needs of the patient and carer at regular intervals (remembering that most problems are progressive).* The first step is building a reminder system into the diary of the electronic record, and the second step is to find the time to utilize it.

9. *Ensured that you have good liaison with any other professionals involved and know who is the key worker.* Make sure you know who is doing what, aim for personal rather than anonymous relationships, try to make joint visits with social workers and old age psychiatrists (a counsel of perfection!).

10. *Arranged to see the carer regularly once the patient dies or is admitted to long-term care.* Because the caring role does not end with the move to a nursing home, or even with death.

11. *Recorded and collated information on the needs of people with dementia and their carers.* This information can be used to guide the commissioning process, but involves more than collecting the data that is easy to audit, and should include the comments and responses of patients and their carers.

The electronic medical record can also be used to support the process of diagnosis, and contribute to problem-solving in managing behavioural problems or reviewing medication use. Decision-support software exists already (see the 6CIT described in Chapter Two), and more is currently being developed which will generate prompts and advice like that shown on the screen images from the Scottish software system GPASS (Figure 6.1).

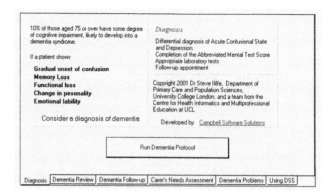

Figure 6.1 GPASS Screenshots

LEARNING ABOUT DEMENTIA

Many primary care professionals will want further training and education to enhance their work with patients with dementia, and with their families. In Figure 6.2 we have summarized the process of dementia care in the community, but to implement this practitioners from all disciplines will need to acquire new knowledge. This knowledge is not going to be acquired passively by listening to lectures from experts in old age psychiatry, neurology or community nursing. Dementia is so complex that learning about it occurs through the experience of solving its problems, including the problem of diagnosis itself, and those organizing professional education on the theme of dementia need to understand how knowledge acquisition occurs (Iliffe, Walters and Rait 2000). How then can practitioners from different disciplines organize their professional development to close the knowledge gaps and skills shortages in dementia care?

There appear to be six important components to any educational process that will change professional practice in a domain as difficult as dementia.

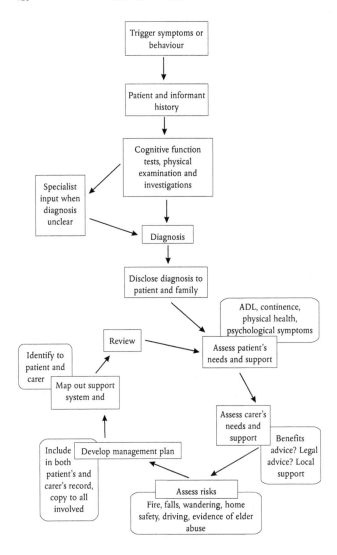

Figure 6.2 The process of dementia care in the community

1. Practitioners must identify their own learning needs, and make the first step towards seeking knowledge (Grant *et al.* 1998). Such awareness of learning needs and motivation to update skills and knowledge is linked to an estimation of expected benefit, both to the practitioners and their patients (Willis and Dubin 1990), which itself depends on recognition of underperformance or lack of knowledge. This approach is the opposite of the type of education in which practitioners opt for topics with which they feel comfortable, and about which they already know much.

2. Learning should be about enhancing performance, emphasizing both the resolution of clinical concerns and better outcomes for patients (Nowlem 1988). In the case of the difficult, complex and sometimes ill-defined problems encountered with dementia, such learning can be viewed as the essence of professionalism (Eraut 2000).

3. Learning needs to be integrated with practice, in terms of convenience, relevance, individualization, self-assessment, interest, speculation about controversial areas, and systematic coverage of the issues (Harden and Laidlaw 1992).

4. Learning should focus on solving problems (Brookfield 1986) and explicitly recognize complexities, uncertainties and conflicting values (Cervero 1988). The more complex the problems to solve, the more realistic can practitioners' 'illness scripts' (templates for disease processes) (Feltovitch and Barrow 1984) become, allowing the accurate allocation of cases to scripts (through pattern recognition) and the enrichment of the scripts as case memory increases

with experience. Empirical evidence supports this model of learning, in that interventions that are multifaceted and that target different barriers to change have been shown to be more effective than single interventions (NHS Centre for Reviews and Dissemination 1999).

5.   Peers and colleagues can be the most effective educators (Nowlem 1988), especially if they use a coaching rather than a didactic approach (Schon 1987). However, there may be limits on who is included as peer or colleague, given the lack of support for multiprofessional learning. Perhaps regrettably, general practitioners seem reluctant to learn with other professionals, although willing to learn from them (Grant and Stanton 2000).

6.   Learning requires a mixture of formal (didactic) and informal (experiential) styles (Durno and Gill 1974; Reedy 1979), corresponding to a mix of propositional (factual) and experiential knowledge (Eraut 2000).

No one learning style suits everybody, and a mixture of methods seems important if clinical practice is to change, but the principles seem clear enough. An evidence-based training programme will have to be based on problem-solving approaches, using case histories that reflect the complexities and problems of real life, if it has a potential for changing clinical practice.

Help is available to support such education and training, and to broaden the base of learning to encompass the different disciplines that have so much to offer in dementia. The growing network of dementia centres have access to the necessary expertise and would make good partners for general practitioners, community nurses or primary care trusts promoting professional development about dementia care. Box 6.1 lists some; if we have missed any out, it was not intentional.

BOX 6.1 DEMENTIA CENTRES

The Dementia Services Development Centres Network

These centres provide services and undertake work across a combination of four core areas: service development; service- and practice-based research; staff training and practice development; information and databases.

Stirling DSDC (Area covered: Scotland)
  University of Stirling, Stirling FK9 4LA. Tel: 01786 467740; fax: 01786 466846
North West Region Dementia Services Research and Development Centre (Area covered: North West England)
  Dover Street Building, University of Manchester, Oxford Road, Manchester M13 9PL. Tel: 0161 275 2000; fax: 0161 275 3924
Dementia North (Area covered: North of England)
  Wolfson Research Centre, Newcastle General Hospital, Westgate Road, Newcastle upon Tyne NE6 4BE. Tel: 0191 256 3318 (general enquiries), 0191 256 3320 (information service): email: dementia.north@ncl.ac.uk
South East England DSDC (under development)
  c/o Invicta Community Care NHS Trust, Priority House, Hermitage Lane, Maidstone ME16 9PH. Tel: 01622 725000 x290; fax: 01622 725290;
  email: equal-invicta@hotmail.com
DSDC Wales
  Cardiff: Service Development Team, Royal Hamadryad Hospital, Hamadryad Road, Cardiff CF10 5UQ. Tel: 029 2049 4952; fax: 029 2049 6431; email: sdteam@cdffcom tr.wales.nhs.uk
Bangor: Neuadd Ardudwy, University of Wales Bangor, Holyhead Road, Bangor L57 2PX. Tel: 01248 383719; fax: 01248 382229; email: dsdc@bangor.ac.uk
Midlands DSDC (under development) (Area covered: West Midlands)
  c/o Social Services Department, Civic Centre, St Peter's

Square, Wolverhampton WV1 1RT. Tel: 01902 555306;
fax: 01902 555361
London DSDC
  University College London, Wolfson Building, 48 Riding
  House Street, London W1N 8AA; email: margot.lindsay@
  ucl.ac.uk
Oxford Dementia Centre
  Headington Hill Hall, Oxford Brookes University,
  Headington, Oxford OX3 0BP. Tel: 01865 484706; fax:
  01865 484919; email: dementia@brookes.ac.uk
Dementia Voice (area covered: South West England)
  Blackberry Hill Hospital, Manor Road, Fishponds, Bristol
  BR16 2EW. Tel: 0117 975 4863; fax: 0117 975 4819;
  e-mail: office@dementiavoice.org.uk
Bradford Dementia Group
  Established by Professor Tom Kitwood in 1992. Following
  the death of Tom Kitwood the leadership of the group was
  taken over by Professor Murna Downs in April 2000. The
  group is a division of the School of Health Studies at the
  University of Bradford and since 1992 has expanded in
  many directions including education, research and training.
  Contact: School of Health Studies, University of Bradford,
  Unity Building, 25 Trinity Road, Bradford BD5 0BB. Tel:
  01274 233996

COMMISSIONING DEMENTIA CARE: THE TRAPS

This book has reviewed good practice in the primary care of
dementia, and we want to encourage that practice to spill over
into the commissioning process for service development.
General practitioners, all groups of primary care nurses and
therapists working in primary care have much to offer from their
experience – and from the evidence growing in their electronic
and written records – that can assist in the process of allocating
resources to services, and stimulating innovation and improvement in care. This may be particularly true for dementia –

because the numbers are relatively small, the illness lasts a long time and involves so many agencies, and the individual stories are so powerful as lessons, accolades and warnings. We hope much of what might be said in the commissioning process is now obvious from the preceding chapters, but we also want to warn against some of the hazards that exist for frail older people in a changing health service environment (Iliffe 1999). Four themes seem important to us: referral as a form of disposal; clinical management as a problem as well as a solution; underutilization of limited resources; and the salience of information.

Referral

The traditional medical model of referral, often seen as a desirable route into accurate diagnosis and appropriate specialist care, can sometimes be a form of disposal of the patient. The general practitioner may relinquish responsibility for patients with dementia, and their families, by referring them to specialist medical services where their needs can be met by the expertise of the multidisciplinary team. But multidisciplinary teams can become overloaded by tasks that could be undertaken by generalists – in particular communication with families, patient and carer support, and provision of information. Similarly, specialist teams and social services may dispose of clients with dementia into under-resourced and under-supported residential care where they are, in effect, warehoused. In these situations referral becomes a one-way valve for the referrer and the referred alike, but it need not be so. Clinical governance requires a search for quality standards, which in dementia care should surely include the basic investigations to exclude treatable causes of dementia, the provision of information about support services to patients and carers, and the organization of supportive follow-up. Specialist expertise relieved of some of the tasks of supporting a growing clientele in the community might become more available to the highest-need groups in residential care, where the quality of life of the patient with dementia, and of their carers, is so easily jeopardized.

Clinical management

'Management' of dementia as a clinical problem places great emphasis on the skills and resources of the managers, but little on the patients and their social support, who become the objects of interventions and the recipients of services. Person-centred approaches that are attractive to professionals and the public alike work against this tendency, but are limited by the resources available and the dominant health service culture of assembly-line processing of patients and problems. Social care may have less of a managerial approach than medicine and nursing and be more enabling, perhaps because its services are rationed and dependent (sometimes over-dependent) upon the efforts of patients and carers. There may be something useful to learn from rationing and the need to limit access to expertise, and specialist teams might do better in the long term to consider themselves more as consultants than managers, using clinical protocols and local training programmes to transfer skills back into general practice where they can be deployed by community and practice nurses as well as doctors. While this has been tried many times in many places, with variable results, it has never before had the benefit of an environment where attention to the quality of services is moving to the centre of the professional stage, as it will with clinical governance and the local authority Best Value programmes.

Underutilisation of resources

Resources are limited, and all professionals argue that more are always needed. However, sometimes they are also underused. Day centre space that is empty for large parts of the week, or skilled staff in residential homes who are not used for training or support of others, constitute a wasted resource. The fact that they could be brought into play if social service budgets were big enough to employ more assessment workers highlights the unreality of the health and social care economy, with money sitting under one budget heading being underspent because of cash limits in another. The pooling of social and health care budgets may solve this, but only if needs are accurately mapped, which brings us back to the commissioning process in primary care groups and trusts.

Information

Patients and carers want information, professionals need information, and so do service planners in the commissioning process. Who then is responsible for collecting and analysing or disseminating such different types of information? Primary care groups and their successor trusts, under both their clinical governance and commissioning responsibilities. Information is required to undertake health and social care needs assessment which includes dispelling the negative stereotyping of dementia care, but who has continuous access to the relevant information for a whole population? Primary care groups, through their practices and clinics. Needs assessment for services for older people includes an assessment of the resources currently available as well as an understanding of how innovative practice developed elsewhere could be introduced and improved upon (Iliffe and Drennan 2000). For example information technology – in the shape of smart housing – could make risk management easier for people with dementia, and for their families and neighbours, and help services to provide more support within their limited resources. Who will be able to commission the necessary development work across agencies? Primary care groups and trusts, with their mix of medical, nursing and social care membership, are close enough to the problems to understand them in detail, and to promote innovative solutions.

The evolution of primary care groups and trusts may be very uneven and difficult, but the opportunities offered for more coherent and effective working for people with dementia are as great as the risks that dementia will remain a low priority for primary care. The input to primary care groups and trusts from social services and community nursing may be crucial to the enhancement of understanding about dementia services, and might also serve an educational role with wider benefits. The primary care group that can map the scale of the dementia burden in its community, the scope and strengths of local services, and introduce the training that will optimise professional inputs will have no problem in tackling other complex, demanding and long-term conditions. In that sense, dementia care can be taken as benchmark against which the development of clinical governance at PCG level can be measured. If this book helps any practitioner in the community to initiate such developments, we will have achieved one of our objectives.

References

Alzheimer's Disease Society (1995) *Right from the Start: Primary Health Care and Dementia.* London: Alzheimer's Disease Society.

Alzheimer's Society (1997) *Experiences of Care in Residential and Nursing Homes: A Survey.* London: Alzheimer's Society.

Aneshensel, C., Pearlin, L., Mullan, J., Zarit, S. and Whitlatch, C. (1995) *Profiles in Care Giving: The Unexpected Career.* San Diego, CA: Academic Press.

Antonelli Incalzi, R., Marra, C., Gemma, A., Capparella, O. and Carbonin, P.U. (1992) 'Unrecognised dementia: Sociodemographic correlates.' *Aging: Clinical and Experimental Research 4,* 327–332.

Bamford, C., Vernon, A., Nicholas, E. and Quereshi, H. (1998) *Outcomes for Older People and Their Carers.* Social Policy Research Unit, University of York.

Baragwanath, A. (1997) 'Bounce and balance: A team approach to risk management for people with dementia living at home.' In M. Marshall (ed) *State of the Art in Dementia Care.* London: Centre for Policy on Ageing.

Barberger-Gateau, P., Dartigues, J-F. and Letenneur, L. (1993) 'Four instrumental activities of daily living score as predictor of one year incident dementia.' *Age and Ageing 22,* 457–463.

Bell, J. and McGregor, I. (1995) 'A challenge to stage theories of dementia.' In Kitwood, T. and Benson, S. (eds) *The New Culture of Dementia Care.* London: Hawker.

Bosanquet, N., May, J. and Johnson, N. (1998) *Alzheimers Disease in the UK: Burden of Disease and Future Care.* Health Policy Review Paper no.12. London: Imperial College of Science, Technology and Medicine.

Bradford Dementia Group (1997) *Evaluating Dementia Care: The DCM Method* (7th edition). Bradford Dementia Group, University of Bradford.

Briggs, R. (1993) 'Comment: Alzheimers disease – your views.' *Geriatric Medicine 23,* 40–41.

Brodaty, H., Howarth, G.C., Mant, A. and Kurrle, S.E. (1994) 'General practice and dementia: A national survey of Australian GPs.' *Medical Journal of Australia 160,* 10–14.

Brooke, P. and Bullock, R. (1999) 'Validation of the 6 item Cognitive Impairment Test.' International Journal of Geriatric Psychiatry 14, 936–940.

Brookfield, S.D. (1986) *Understanding and Facilitating Adult Learning.* Buckingham: Open University Press.

Brotzman, G.L. and Butler, D.J. (1991) 'Cross cultural issues in the disclosure of a terminal diagnosis: A case study.' *Journal of Family Practice 32*, 426–427.

Buck, D., Gregson, B.A. and Bamford, C.H. (1997) 'Psychological distress among informal supporters of frail older people at home and in institutions.' *International Journal of Geriatric Psychiatry 12*, 737–744.

Burns, A., Russell, E. and Page, S. (1999) 'New drugs for Alzheimer's disease.' *British Journal of Psychiatry 174*, 476–479.

Cameron, K. and Chapman, A. (eds) (2000) *CarenapD: Care Needs Assessment Pack for Dementia*. Dementia Services Development Centre, University of Stirling.

Carers National Association (1996) *Who Cares? Perceptions of Caring and Carers*. London: Carers National Association.

Caring Costs Alliance (1996) *The True Cost of Caring: A Survey of Carers' Lost Income*. London: Caring Costs Alliance.

Centre for Policy on Ageing (1996) *A Better Home Life: A Code of Good Practice in Residential and Nursing Home Care*. London: Centre for Policy on Ageing.

Cervero, R.M. (1988) *Effective Continuing Education for Professionals*. San Francisco, CA: Jossey-Bass.

Chenoweth, B. and Spencer, B. (1986) 'Dementia: The experience of family caregivers.' *Gerontologist 26*, 267–272.

Clarke, C. (1999) 'Dementia care partnerships.' In T. Adams and C. Clarke C (eds) *Dementia Care: Developing Partnerships in Practice*. London: Baillière Tindall.

Cohen, D., Kennedy, G. and Eisdorfer, C. (1985) 'Phases of change in the patient with Alzheimer's disease.' *Journal of the American Geriatric Society 32*, 11–15.

Cottrell, V. and Schulz, R. (1993) 'The perspective of the patient with Alzheimer's disease: A neglected dimension of dementia research.' *Gerontologist 33*, 205–211.

Dawson, S. (1992) *Analysing Organisations*. London: Macmillan Press.

De Lepeleire, J. and Heyrman, J. (1999) 'Diagnosis and management of dementia in primary care at an early stage: The need for a new concept and an adapted structure.' *Theoretical Medicine and Bioethics 20*, 215–228.

De Lepeleire, J., Heyrman, J., Baro, F., Buntinx, F. and Lasuy, C. (1994) 'How do general practitioners diagnose dementia?' *Family Practice 11*, 148–152.

De Lepeleire, J., Heyrman, J. and Buntinx, F. (1998) 'The early diagnosis of dementia: Triggers, early signs and luxating events.' *Family Practice 15*, 431–436.

De Lepeleire J., Heyrman, J. and Buntinx, F. (1999) 'The development of an instrument for the diagnosis of dementia in general practice.' Paper presented at the WONCA Conference, Mallorca, May.

Department of Health (2000) *The National Strategy for Carers*. London: The Stationery Office. http://www.carers.gov.uk

Downs, M. (1997) 'The emergence of the person in dementia research.' *Ageing and Society 17*, 597–607.

Dura, J.R., Stukenberg, K.W. and Kiecolt-Glaser, J.K. (1991) 'Anxiety and depressive disorders in adult children caring for demented parents.' *Psychology and Ageing 6*, 467–473.

Durno, D. and Gill, M. (1974) 'Survey of general practitioners' views on postgraduate education in north east Scotland.' *Journal of the Royal College of General Practitioners 24*, 648–654.

Eccles, M., Clarke, J., Livingston, M., Freemantle, N. and Mason, J. (1998) 'North of England evidence based guidelines development project: Guideline for the primary care management of dementia.' *British Medical Journal 317*, 802–808.

Eefsting, J.A., Boersma, F., van den Brink, W. and van Tilburg, W. (1996) 'Differences in the prevalence of dementia based on community survey and general practitioner recognition.' *Psychological Medicine 26*, 1223–1230.

Ellis, P.M. and Tattersall, M.H. (1999) 'How should doctors communicate the diagnosis of cancer to patients?' *Ann Med 31*, 336–341.

Eraut, M. (2000) *Developing Professional Knowledge and Competence.* London: Falmer.

Escobar, J., Burnham, A., Karno, M., Forsyth, A., Landsverk, J. and Golding, J. (1986) 'Use of the MMSE in a community population of mixed ethnicity.' *Journal of Nervous and Mental Disease 174*, 607–614.

Feltovitch, P.J. and Barrow, H.S. (1984) 'Issues of generality in medical problem solving.' In H.G. Schmidt and M.L. de Volder (eds) *Tutorials in Problem-based Learning.* Van Gorcum, Assen.

Finch, H. (2000) 'When relatives care.' *Journal of Dementia Care 8*, 14.

Flicker, C., Ferris, S. and Reisberg, B. (1993) 'A longditudinal study of cognitive function in elderly persons with subjective memory complaints.' *JAGS 41*, 1029–32.

Fortinsky, R. and Wasson, J. (1997) 'How do physicians diagnose dementia? Evidence from clinical vignette responses.' *American Journal of Alzheimer's Disease 12*, 51–61.

Fruin, D. (1998) *A Matter of Chance for Carers: Inspection of Local Authority Support for Carers.* Social Care Group reference number CI(98)19. London: Department of Health.

Gallo, J., Franch, M. and Reichel, W. (1991) 'Dementing illness: The patient, caregiver and community.' *American Family Physician 43*, 1668–1675.

Glosser, G., Wexler, D. and Balmelli, M. (1985) 'Physicians' and familes' perspectives on the medical management of dementia.' *Journal of the American Geriatric Society 33*, 383–391.

Goldsmith, M. (1996) *Hearing the Voice of People with Dementia.* London: Jessica Kingsley Publishers.

Goodchild, C. (1999) 'Speaking up: Advocacy for people with dementia.' *Journal of Dementia Care 7*, 619.

Grant, G. and Nolan, M. (1993) 'Informal carers: Sources and concomitants of satisfaction.' *Health and Social Care 1*, 147–159.

Grant, J. and Stanton, F. (2000) *The Effectiveness of Continuing Professional Development*. Edinburgh: The Association for the Study of Medical Education.

Grant, J., Stanton, F., Flood, S., Mack, J. and Waring, C. (1998) *An Evaluation of Educational Needs and Provision for Doctors within Three Years of Completion of Training*. London: Joint Centre for Education in Medicine.

Gray, A. and Fenn, P. (1993) 'Alzheimer's disease: The burden of the illness in England.' *Health Trends 25*, 31–37.

Haley, W., Clair, J. and Saulsberry, K. (1992) 'Family caregiver satisfaction with the medical care of their demented relatives.' *Gerontologist 32*, 219–226.

Harden, R.M. and Laidlaw, J.M. (1992) 'Effective continuing education: The CRISIS criteria.' *Medical Education 26*, 408–422.

Henwood, M. (1998) *Ignored and Invisible? Carer Experience of the NHS*. London: Carers National Association.

Hofman, A., Rocca, W., Brayne, C., Breteler, M., Clarke, M., Cooper, B. *et al.* (1991) 'The prevalence of dementia in Europe: A collaborative study of 1980–1990 findings.' *International Journal of Epidemiology 20*, 736–748.

Holzhausen, E. and Pearlman, V. (2000) *Caring on the Breadline*. London: Carers National Association.

Horsley, S., Barrow, S., Gent, N. and Astbury, J. (1998) 'Informal care and psychiatric morbidity.' *Journal of Public Health Medicine 20*, 180–185.

Iliffe, S. (1999) 'Commissioning dementia care: A strategy emerges?' *Journal of Dementia Care 7*, 3, 14–15.

Iliffe, S. and Drennan, V. (2000) *Primary Care for Older People*. Oxford General Practice Series 44. Oxford: Oxford University Press.

Iliffe, S. and Lenihan, P. (2000) *Innovative Primary Care for Older People*. London: Department of Primary Care and Population Sciences, Royal Free and UCL Medical School.

Iliffe, S., Haines, A., Gallivan, S. *et al.* (1990) 'Screening for cognitive impairment using the mini-mental state examination.' *British Journal of General Practice 40*, 277–279.

Iliffe, S., Mitchley, S., Gould, M. and Haines, A. (1991) 'Evaluation of the use of brief screening instruments for dementia, depression and problem drinking among elderly people in general practice.' *British Journal of General Practice 44*, 503–507.

Iliffe, S., Walters, K. and Rait, G. (2000) 'Shortcomings in the care of dementia in general practice: Towards an educational strategy.' *Aging and Mental Health 4*, 286–291.

Ireichen, B. (1994) 'Managing demented old people in the community: a review.' *Family Practice 11*, 210–215.

Jagger, C., Clarke, M., Anderson, J. and Battock, T. (1992) 'Misclassification of dementia by the mini-mental state examination – Are education and social class the only factors?' *Age and Ageing 21*, 404–411.

Keady, J. (1997) 'Maintaining involvement: A meta concept to describe the dynamics of dementia.' In M. Marshall (ed) *State of the Art in Dementia Care.* London: Centre for Policy on Ageing.

Kings Fund (1986) *Living Well into Old Age: Applying Principles of Good Practice to Services for People with Dementia.* Project Paper no 63. London: Kings Fund Centre.

Kirmayer, L. (1989) 'Variations in the response to psychiatric disorders and emotional distress.' *Social Science and Medicine 29*, 327–339.

Kitwood, T. (1997) *Dementia Reconsidered: The Person Comes First.* Buckingham: Open University Press.

Kitwood, T. and Bredin, K. (1992) *Person to Person: A Guide to the Care of Those with Failing Mental Powers* (2nd edition). Loughton, Essex: Gale Centre Publications.

Lagay, A., van der Meij, J. and Hijmans, W. (1992) 'Validation of medical history taking as part of a population based survey in subjects aged 85 and over.' *British Medical Journal 304*, 1091–1093.

Levin, E., Sinclair, I. and Gorbach, P. (1989) *Families, Confusion and Old Age.* Aldershot: Gower.

Lintern, T., Woods, B. and Phair, L. (2000) 'Training is not enough to change care practice.' *Journal of Dementia Care 8*, 2, 15–16.

Maguire, C.P., Kirby, M., Coen, R. *et al.* (1996) 'Family members' attitudes toward telling the patient with Alzheimer's disease their diagnosis.' *British Medical Journal 313*, 529–530.

Malone, C. and Mackenzie, R. (2000) 'Community care: In the know.' *Health Service Journal 110*, 5721, 28–29.

McGeer, P.L. (2000) 'Cyclo-oxygenase 2 inhibitors: Rationale and therapeutic potential for Alzheimer's disease.' *Drugs and Ageing 17*, 1–11.

McShane, R., Keene, J., Gedling, C., Fairburn, C., Jacoby, R. and Hope, T. (1997) 'Do neuroleptic drugs hasten cognitive decline in dementia?' *British Medical Journal 314*, 266–270.

Melzer, D., Hopkins, S., Pencheon, D. *et al.* (1994) *Dementia in Health Care Needs Assessment: The Epidemiologically Based Needs Assessment Reviews.* Oxford: Radcliffe Medical Press.

Morgan, D. and Zhao, P. (1993) 'The doctor–caregiver relationship: Managing the care of family members with Alzheimer's disease.' *Qualitative Health Research 3*, 133–164.

Moriarty, J. and Webb, S. (2000) *Part of Their Lives: Community Care for Older People with Dementia.* Bristol: The Policy Press.

Murray, J., Schenider, J., Banerjee, S. and Mann, R. (1999) 'Eurocare: A cross national study of co-resident spouse carers for people with Alzheimer's disease – A qualitative analysis of the experience of care giving.' *International Journal of Geriatric Psychiatry 14*, 662–667.

Newens, A.J., Forster, D.F. and Kay, D.W. (1994) 'Referral patterns and diagnosis on presenile Alzheimers disease: Implications for general practice.' *British Journal of General Practice 44*, 405–407.

NHS Centre for Reviews and Dissemination. (1999) *Effective Health Care: Getting Evidence into Practice*, Volume 5 (1). York: University of York.

North of England Evidence Based Guidelines Project (1998) *The Primary Care Management of Dementia*. Department of Primary Care and the Centre for Health Services Research, University of Newcastle upon Tyne.

Nowlem, P.M. (1988) *A New Approach to Continuing Education for Business and the Professions*. New York: Macmillan.

Nurock, S. (2000) 'GPs we need you!' *Journal of Dementia Care 8*, 5, 26–27.

O'Connor, D., Pollitt, P., Brook, C.P.B. and Reiss, B. (1989) 'The validity of informant studies histories in a community study of dementia.' *International Journal of Geriatric Psychiatry 4*, 203–208.

O'Connor, D., Pollitt, P., Hyde, J., Reiss, B. and Roth, M. (1988) 'Do general practitioners miss dementia in elderly patients?' *British Medical Journal 297*, 1107–1110.

Office for National Statistics (1998) *Informal Carers*. London: The Stationery Office.

Olafsdottir, M. and Marcusson, J. (1996) 'Diagnosis of dementia at the primary care level.' *Acta Neurologica Scandinavica 165*, S58–S62.

Pointon, B. (2000) 'So we all shed a tear. Now what?' Alzheimers Society UK Newsletter January 2000.

Pollitt, P. (1996) 'Dementia in old age: An anthropological perspective.' *Psychological Medicine 26*, 1061–1074.

Rait, G. and Burns, A. (1998) 'Screening for depression and cognitive impairment in older people from ethnic minority backgrounds.' *Age and Ageing 27*, 271–275.

Rait, G., Burns, A. and Chew, C. (1996) 'Age, ethnicity and mental illness: A triple whammy?' *British Medical Journal 313*, 1347–1348.

Reedy, B. (1979) *General Practitioners and Postgraduate Education in the Northern Region*. Occasional Paper 9. London: Royal College of General Practitioners.

Royal Commission on Long Term Care (1999) *With Respect to Old Age: Long Term Care – Rights and Responsibilities*. Cm 4192–1. London: The Stationery Office.

Rubin, S.M., Glasser, M.L. and Werckle, M.A. (1987) 'The examination of physicians' awareness of dementing disorders.' *Journal of the American Geriatric Society 35*, 1051–1058.

Russo, J. and Vitaliano, P.P. (1995) 'Life events as correlates of burden in spouse caregivers of persons with Alzheimer's disease.' *Experimental Ageing Research 21*, 273–294.

Schiff, R., Rajkumar, C. and Bulpitt, C. (2000) 'Views of elderly people on living wills: Interview study.' *British Medical Journal 320*, 1640–1641.

Schneider, J., Kavanagh, S., Knapp, M., Beecham, J. and Netten, A. (1993) 'Elderly people with advanced cognitive impairment in England: Resource use and costs.' *Ageing and Society 13*, 27–50.

Schneider, L.S., Pollock, V.E. and Lyness, S.A. (1990) 'A meta-analysis of controlled trials of neuroleptic treatment in dementia.' *Journal of the American Geriatric Society 38*, 553–563.

Schon, D. (1987) *Educating the Reflective Practitioner.* San Francisco, CA: Jossey-Bass.

Shapiro, S., German, P., Skinner, E., Vonkorff, M., Turner, R., Klein, L. *et al.* (1987) 'An experiment to change detection and management of mental morbidity in primary care.' *Medical Care 25*, 327–339.

Sloper, P. and Turner, S. (1993) 'Determinants of parental satisfaction with disclosure of disability.' *Developmental Medicine and Child Neurology 35*, 816–825.

Social Services Inspectorate (1993) *No Longer Afraid: The Safeguarding of Older People in Domestic Settings.* HMSO, London.

Social Services Inspectorate (1996) *Assessing Older People Living with Dementia in the Community: Practice Issues for Social and Health Services.* Social Services Inspectorate/Department of Health.

Social Services Inspectorate (1997) *At Home with Dementia: Inspection of Services for Older People with Dementia in the Community.* Social Services Inspectorate/Department of Health.

Thompson, C. and Spilsbury, K. (2001) 'Support for carers of people with Alzheimer's-type disease.' In the Cochrane Library: Cochrane collaboration, Issue 3. Oxford: Update Software.

Toner, H. (1992) 'What do we mean by assessment?' In D. Haxby (ed) *Dementia: Diagnosis and Assessment.* Stirling: Dementia Services Development Centre.

Twigg, J. (1989) 'Models of carers: How do social care agencies conceptualise their relationships with informal carers?' *Journal of Social Policy 18*, 53–66.

Twigg, J. and Atkin, K. (1994) *Carers Perceived – Policy and Practice in Informal Care.* Buckingham: Open University Press.

van Hout, H. (1999) *Diagnosing Dementia: Evaluation of the Clinical Practice of General Practitioners and a Memory Clinic.* University of Nijmegen.

Vassilas, C.A. and Donaldson, J. (1999) 'Few GPs tell patients of their diagnosis of Alzheimer's disease.' *British Medical Journal 318*, 536.

Verhey, F., Ponds, R., Rozendal, N. and Jilles, J. (1995) 'Depression, insight and personality changes in Alzheimers disease and vascular dementia.' *Journal of Geriatric Psychiatry and Neurology 8*, 23–27.

142   PRIMARY CARE AND DEMENTIA

Victor, C. (1997) *Community Care and Older People.* Cheltenham: Stanley Thornes Publishers.

Willis S.L. and Dubin, S.S. (1990) *Maintaining Professional Competence.* San Francisco, CA: Jossey-Bass.

Wimo, A., Ljunggren, G. and Winblad, B. (1997) 'Costs of dementia and dementia care: A review.' *International Journal of Geriatric Psychiatry 12,* 841–856.

Wolff, L.E. (1994) 'Do general practitioners and old age psychiatrists differ in their attitudes to dementia?' *International Journal of Geriatric Psychiatry 10,* 63–69.

Subject Index

146

PRIMARY CARE AND DEMENTIA

Dementia Voice 130
denial 61, 63, 64, 95
depersonalization 106
depression 13–15, 25, 28, 33, 34, 42,
    64, 68, 75, 77, 82, 92, 94, 95, 100
    acute confusion and dementia,
      differentiating 16–24
desires 62
diabetes 21, 29, 45
diagnosing dementia 25–33
    after diagnosis 47–58
    confirming and conveying 35–59
    delayed 27–30
    diagnostic process 36–46
    disclosing 47–52
    good practice 122
    how should diagnosis be given? 50–2
    summary of (flow chart) 28
diarrhoea 58
diet 56
direct care provision 56
disability living allowance 92
disempowerment 104
disinhibition 13, 15, 31, 62, 66
disorientation 14, 15, 18, 23
district nurse/nursing team 13, 63, 65,
    73, 77, 116
diuretics 75
dizziness 58
Donepezil 58
dressing 56
driving 82, 84
drowsiness 23
drug(s)
    known to cause confusion 29
    toxicity 18
    see also medication
DSDC see Dementia Services
    Development Centres Network
DSDC Wales 129
DVLA 84
dysphasia 15, 16, 76

early dementia 29–30, 33, 34, 50
eating, irregular 73
economic impact of caring for someone
    with dementia 91–2
economics, family 32
education 30, 31, 36, 106, 121–2, 125
electrolyte imbalance 75, 76
emotional changes/problems 13, 15, 30,
    33, 55
emotional support for carers 96
emotions, effect of progressing dementia
    on 102
empathy 100
energy 62
    loss of 20, 33, 64
enlarged prostate 12
environmental health 113
epileptiform seizures 16
ethnicity 30
ethnic minorities 30
evaluating quality of care for people with
    dementia 113–15
excluding uncommon causes of dementia
    44–6
expressive dysphasia 15, 16
extracellular degenerative plaques 24

faecal incontinence 69, 76
falls 25
'false positive' diagnoses 43
family 43, 45, 47, 49, 54, 57, 60, 62, 66,
    96
    economics 32
    members as carers 13, 32, 61, 79–81,
      86–7, 89, 101
      and professionals, problems between
        90
fatigue 18, 58
fear of dementia 32
fearfulness 18
features of dementia at different points in
    its path 15–16
feelings 62
fidgeting 66

Name Index

CPI Antony Rowe
Chippenham, UK
2018-12-04 11:39